WHAT TO DO WHEN THE DOCTOR SAYS IT'S

Rheumatoid Arthritis

WHAT TO DO WHEN THE DOCTOR SAYS IT'S

Rheumatoid Arthritis

Cure Your Pain, Become More Active,
and Take Control of Your Medical Care

HARRY D. FISCHER, M.D. AND WINNIE YU

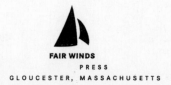

FAIR WINDS
PRESS
GLOUCESTER, MASSACHUSETTS

Text © 2005 by Harry D. Fischer, M.D. and Winnie Yu

First published in the USA in 2005 by
Fair Winds Press
33 Commercial Street
Gloucester, MA 01930

09 08 07 06 05 1 2 3 4 5

ISBN 1-59233-146-7

Library of Congress Cataloging-in-Publication Data available

Original cover design by Laura Shaw Design
Book design by *tabula rasa* graphic design

Printed and bound in USA

The information in this book is for educational purposes only. It is not intended to replace the advice of a physician or medical practitioner. Please see your health care provider before beginning any new health program.

To Jeff —WY

To my wife, Elisa and children—Pamela, Douglas, and Travis —HF

A Note to Readers

Shortly before the book went to press, Bextra, a COX-2 inhibitor, was removed from the market, at the request of the U.S. Food and Drug Administration. The move came on the heels of Merck's withdrawal of Vioxx, another COX-2 that appeared to be associated with cardiovascular problems, including heart attack and stroke.

The FDA has required strongly worded labeling on Celebrex, the remaining COX-2 painkiller, and other prescription-strength NSAIDs. The labels will highlight the potential for increased risk of cardiovascular events and gastrointestinal bleeding associated with their use. In the meantime, as a physician I am exercising extra caution in prescribing these medications, especially for patients at high risk for cardiovascular problems. All patients should thoroughly discuss the use of any medications with their doctors.

—H.D.F.

CONTENTS

ACKNOWLEDGMENTS

I'd like to thank my editor, Donna Raskin, who entrusted me with a subject as complex as rheumatoid arthritis. I'd also like to express my appreciation to the behind-the-scenes people at Fair Winds Press—Rhiannon Soucy and Brigid Carroll, among them—the unsung editorial heroes who work so hard to bring important topics like RA to light and who do it with so little recognition.

In addition, I want to acknowledge and remember my original collaborator, Dr. Oscar Gluck, whose initial enthusiasm and energy for this project was tragically cut short by his sudden and unexpected death. In his place stepped the wonderful Dr. Harry Fischer, who has given so generously of his time, wisdom, and experience. His patients are blessed to have him as a partner and health-care provider in their struggles against all rheumatological illnesses, not just RA.

I must also thank all the people who were profiled in the book, who took the time to talk to me about their experiences with RA. They are remarkable people, facing a challenging and unpredictable illness and doing it with amazing grace despite the pain. It is through their experiences that I hope readers will find their own courage and strength.

Finally, I must extend my gratitude to my family—Jeff, Samantha, and Annie—for their endless love, support, and patience. And special thanks go out to my mother and mother-in-law, whose babysitting services help make all my writing efforts possible.

—W.Y.

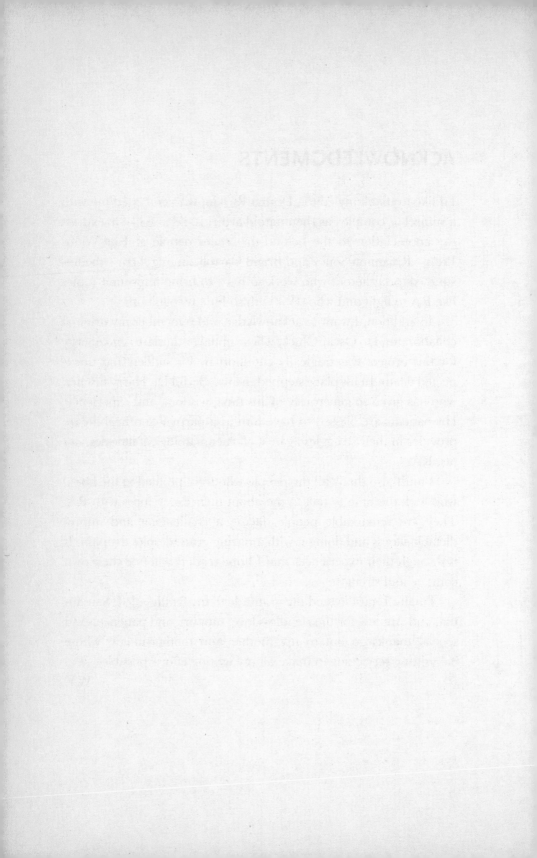

INTRODUCTION

My interest in rheumatology and rheumatoid arthritis began during my residency in internal medicine twenty-five years ago. Training at a hospital that was affiliated with an orthopedic/rheumatology specialty hospital allowed me the opportunity to spend one month during each of my three years of residency caring for patients with rheumatic diseases. Most of my early knowledge and understanding of this disease came from treating hospitalized patients with rheumatoid arthritis. At this time, patients newly diagnosed with the disease could be hospitalized to initiate evaluation and treatment. Simply placing a patient in the hospital was considered a form of treatment. Today, rheumatology has evolved into an outpatient specialty with hospitalization being reserved only for the rare complications of the disease or for surgery. Over the past twenty years not only has there been a dramatic change in the role of the hospital but also in the treatments available.

In the early 1980s, following my residency, I became a fellow in rheumatology. At that time, patients with rheumatoid arthritis were treated with both anti-inflammatory medication as well as immunosuppressive agents. While large doses of aspirin—"aspirin meals" of four to five aspirins four times a day—were still being used, newer anti-inflammatory medications were becoming the mainstay of therapy. These agents had longer half-lives. They were also considerably more convenient and needed to be taken only once or twice a day.

Immune suppressants were nothing new. The use of medications that suppress the immune system had begun decades earlier with the introduction of cortisone in 1949. Cortisone had such a dramatic and profound effect on the manifestations of rheumatoid arthritis that a Nobel Prize was awarded for its use in this condition. However, by the time of my fellowship, the many problems associated with long-term cortisone use were well recognized, and its use was falling into disfavor.

Newer medications that suppressed the immune system differently than cortisone did were becoming more widely used in the treatment of rheumatoid arthritis. However, these medications left much to be desired. Both the anti-inflammatory and immunosuppressive agents that came into use were very nonspecific in their effects. While they did produce some desired effects, many nondesired effects were also seen. I was taught that our use of these medications represented a "sledgehammer" approach to the treatment of rheumatoid arthritis.

Fortunately, much has changed in the past decade. Scientists have made great strides in their understanding of the biologic mechanisms that cause inflammation. They've also made a similar leap in their knowledge of the immune mechanisms underlying rheumatoid arthritis. With this new knowledge, they've developed medications that can specifically target abnormalities found in patients with rheumatoid arthritis. They have made significant progress in modifying the "sledgehammer" approach. Until recently, scientists believed that the new medications being used to treat rheumatoid arthritis were safer, more specific, and more effective.

Unfortunately, sometimes things do not turn out exactly as expected. Concerns have been raised about the newer anti-inflammatory medications once touted as "super aspirins." Similarly, the newer immunosuppressive agents and biologic therapies have been found to create new problems not previously seen. While great strides have been made, clearly there is a continued need for newer therapies.

Despite these advancements and setbacks, I am convinced that today, when compared to when I first became a doctor, patients with rheumatoid arthritis are living more productive and pain-free lives than ever before. I was reminded of this a few weeks ago. While I was walking along Broadway in New York City, a car pulled over to the sidewalk as its driver honked the horn. Out bounded one of the first patients I had ever seen with rheumatoid arthritis. As a medical resident, I had cared for him during a prolonged hospitalization shortly after his diagnosis. He had clearly come a long way since the early days of his disease. Following many different trials of medications and several surgeries, he was doing quite well.

It is my expectation that over the next few years, there will be an even greater understanding of the causes and mechanisms involved in the development of rheumatoid arthritis. These advances will likely lead to more effective treatments and possibly even a cure.

—*Dr. Harry D. Fischer*

CHAPTER ONE ❧

What Is Rheumatoid Arthritis?

Every day, millions of people awaken to aches and pains in their joints. Their fingers feel stiff and painful. Their feet are achy, maybe swollen. Their knees may creak and be difficult to bend.

For the vast majority of these people, the aches are the result of wear and tear brought on by the destruction of cartilage in bone that occurs over time and with age.

But for others, the aches and pain are the result of an insidious internal assault of the immune system on the body's joints. These people have rheumatoid arthritis.

In short, rheumatoid arthritis (RA) is an autoimmune disease that causes inflammation in the lining of the joints. When a person has an autoimmune disease, the immune system mistakenly attacks the cells, tissues, and organs of his or her own body. In the case of RA, it attacks the lining of the joints, resulting in a decrease in the range of motion in the affected joints, as well as swelling, pain, and a feeling of warmth. Left uncontrolled and in rare cases, the disease can spread elsewhere and affect major organs.

RA derives its name from the body parts if afflicts. As a rheumatic disorder, RA is a connective tissue disease characterized by inflammation and/or pain in the muscles, joints, or fibrous tissue, namely the body's supportive framework and organs. Other rheumatic conditions include lupus, scleroderma, and fibromyalgia. RA is also one of more than 100 forms of arthritis, a term that refers to conditions in which the joints become inflamed. Osteoarthritis, the most common form, results from the wear and tear that can occur over time. Other forms of arthritis include gout, ankylosing spondylitis, and juvenile rheumatoid arthritis.

Approximately 1 percent of the U.S. population, or 2.1 million people, have RA. Most of these people are women. In fact, the number of women who have RA exceeds the number of men by three to one. Many people with RA are initially diagnosed between the ages of thirty and fifty-five. The disease occurs in all races and ethnic groups and can begin in childhood and young adulthood. The prevalence is slightly higher among Pima and Chippewa Indians and slightly lower among African-Americans living in rural settings. The incidence of RA generally increases with age.

Unlike osteoarthritis, RA is not a degenerative condition. Rather it is an autoimmune disorder, much like Type 1 diabetes, lupus, scleroderma, and multiple sclerosis—all conditions in which a malfunction in the immune system causes the body to turn on itself and attack healthy tissue. Why this occurs in RA—or in any of these conditions for that matter—is a subject of intense study but remains an unsolved medical mystery.

If you've just learned that you have rheumatoid arthritis, then you are already familiar with the aches and pain it can cause. You may already be experiencing a reduction in your range of motion. You may be plagued by persistent fatigue or a low-grade fever. You may be feeling frustrated, even depressed, over the limitations it's imposing on your life.

What you may not know, however, is that the lifestyle choices you make, as well as the treatment regimen you choose, can have a tremendous impact on your health and well-being and how well you live with RA. Only by becoming better educated about RA will you gain some control over this disease.

ANATOMY OF A HEALTHY JOINT

The fingers. The shoulders. The knees. Two bones meet at the important joint, a natural wonder of engineering. When we grab a utensil, walk up a staircase, or reach down to retrieve a dropped object, these joints bend and flex, allowing us to move through space and to perform our tasks. Some joints move like the hinge of a door, such as your fingers or knees. Others, including the wrist and ankle, can move in many different directions. Still other joints, such as the shoulder and hip, have a ball-in-socket structure that allows for movement in many directions. In all, we have about seventy movable joints in our bodies.

At the end of each bone is a covering called cartilage. Behaving like a cushion, cartilage keeps the bones from rubbing against each other and gives the joint its smooth flexibility. Cartilage is made up of cells called chrondrocytes and surrounded in a framework of connective tissue called collagen.

Surrounding the entire joint is a joint capsule, which is lined with a type of tissue called synovium. The synovium, also called the synovial membrane, is a thin layer of cells that produces synovial fluid. The fluid acts as a lubricant for the joint, nourishing the cartilage and bones inside the joint capsule and allowing the joint to move smoothly. Connecting the two bones of a joint is the ligament.

The joint is also supported by muscles and tendons. Muscles give joints the strength to move. Different muscles allow the same joint to move in different directions. Think of the way your shoulder joint moves as you reach across your chest, over your head, or behind your neck. Muscles also provide the stability needed to hold a joint in position. Even something as simple as standing requires muscles to sustain the joints in the knees and hips.

Muscles are attached to bones by tendons, which in turn are housed in tendon sheaths. Like the synovium of the joint, the tendon sheath encases the tendon, allowing it to glide smoothly. Other structures that help facilitate smooth muscle movement are bursae, sacs located between or under muscles. Bursae shield the joint and muscle from friction as well as from external pressure.

In healthy people, the joint functions like a well-orchestrated machine, supporting, lubricating, and nourishing the bones and muscles as they perform tasks and movements throughout the day, often without even a moment's thought from you. But in people who develop RA, these parts can be affected, even destroyed, and movement of the joint becomes challenging, if not impossible.

WHEN RA ATTACKS

As we've already mentioned, RA is caused by an abnormal autoimmune response in which the body attacks itself, in this case targeting the joints. The immune system is an intricate and critical part of the body that protects us from infection and disease. In healthy people, the body summons white blood cells whenever it is confronted by foreign invaders, such as bacteria or viruses (which are called antigens). The cells gather at the site of the invasion and work together to destroy the invading organism and bring about healing.

In a person with RA, these white blood cells are mysteriously summoned for no reason, and they begin to produce antibodies against cells and tissues that are in your body. When the immune system mistakenly identifies its own cells as foreign, it is called an autoimmune response. In RA, these overactive white blood cells travel to the synovium, where they start to attack the healthy cells there. The attack causes inflammation, swelling, redness, and warmth—in short, producing the symptoms of RA.

The white blood cells involved in an RA attack are varied and distinct. Below are four of the key players:

Neutrophils, also called polymorphonuclear leukocytes, make up the bulk of our white blood cells. These inflammatory white blood cells engulf and destroy antigens. In people with RA, the neutrophils leave the blood vessels, travel through the synovium, and settle in the synovial fluid, where they promote inflammation.

Macrophages play several roles in the immune system. They ingest and destroy cell debris, bacterial invaders, and diseased cells. They also release chemicals that lure other white blood cells to the scene of a perceived invasion by an antigen and present the invaders to lymphocytes, white blood cells with distinct roles in the immune system.

In doing their tasks, macrophages produce substantial amounts of cytokines, chemicals that allow components of the immune system to communicate with one another. As you will read later, two of these cytokines, tumor necrosis factor (TNF) and interleukin-1, have come under intense scrutiny for their pivotal role in promoting inflammation. They have also become a major focus for new treatments for RA.

These chemical messengers perpetuate the growth of blood vessels going to the synovium, which in turn causes the joint to feel warm. When cytokines leak into the bloodstream, they bring on the fatigue that is almost always a symptom of RA. Cytokines are also responsible for the production of prostaglandins and leukotrienes, substances that promote pain and inflammation.

T cell lymphocytes also contribute to the release of cytokines. Working along with macrophages, T lymphocytes cause the synovial cells to multiply abnormally, significantly increasing the bulk of the synovium by 20 to 100 times its normal size.

T lymphocytes come in several varieties and are major players in the immune reaction. Helper T cells work by alerting B cell lymphocytes to produce antibodies to fight off foreign invaders.

Suppressor T cells shut down immune function. Killer T cells, also called cytotoxic T cells, recognize, attack, and destroy antigens. In people with RA, the most common T cells are the Th1 helper cells, which promote inflammation.

B cell lymphocytes are specialized white blood cells that churn out antibodies, the actual proteins that neutralize and destroy antigens. The B lymphocytes can produce antibodies on their own in direct response to an antigen or may be summoned by the T cells. In people who have RA, these B lymphocytes may produce an abundance of one particular antibody called rheumatoid factor.

As the disease progresses, these antibodies hook up with antigens and become covered in a layer of immune system proteins called complements. These immune complexes, as they are called, become clumps of sticky proteins that form deposits within the joint and attract more white blood cells, thereby causing even more inflammation.

Under attack, the joint becomes swollen, red, and warm. This inflammation of the synovium is called synovitis and results in a great deal of pain. During inflammation, the synovial cells grow and divide abnormally, causing the synovium to become thick and swollen and puffy to the touch. The synovial membrane, once thin, is now considerably thickened into a mass called a pannus.

Over time, these abnormal synovial cells begin to invade and destroy the cartilage and bone within the joint. Doctors now agree that most of the damage to the bone occurs in the first two years of the disease, which is why early and aggressive treatment has become so critical in treating the disease. The invasion eventually weakens the muscles, ligaments, and tendons surrounding the joint, making it hard for the joint to perform its function.

In some cases, RA will travel to other parts of the body, and the joint pain may spread. Some patients may experience dry eyes and mouth, anemia, and neck pain. In extreme but rare cases, the disease can cause inflammation in the nerves, the lining of the lungs, or the sac around the heart.

SIGNS AND SYMPTOMS

The internal attack on the joints by the patient's own immune system causes a constellation of symptoms that varies greatly from one person to the next. For some people, the symptoms linger for months, even years, before patients ever even suspect they have RA. They pass off the achy joints as a sign of old age, and the fatigue as a sign of having too much to do. Other patients, however, may experience severe cases that come on suddenly and advance quickly. This great variability of symptoms from one patient to the next is, in fact, a hallmark of RA.

RA does tend to involve specific joints, including the metacarpophalangeal (MCP) joints, which are the first row of knuckles down from the wrist, and the proximal interphalangeal (PIP) joints, which are the second row of joints. The first row of joints on the toes down from the ankle, called the metatarsophalangeal (MTP) joints, may also be affected.

Pain and stiffness in these joints is also common in other rheumatic diseases, such as lupus and scleroderma. And by themselves, these symptoms are not indicative of RA. But in people who have RA, the pain tends to occur symmetrically, meaning that if you have stiffness in a joint on the left hand, you'll also have it in the same joint on the right. In some patients, the joints in the shoulders, knees, elbows, or wrists are involved.

Another common symptom of RA is morning stiffness or stiffness occurring after prolonged periods of inactivity. While many people may awaken feeling a bit stiff, people who have RA experience morning stiffness that often lasts an hour or more.

Approximately a third of RA patients develop rheumatoid nodules. These tiny nodules develop below the skin and vary in size from that of a tiny grain to that of a golf ball. These nodules are not attached to anything but are free-floating lumps usually found in the back of the elbow. They also occur on the front of the knee, the hands, and other pressure points, including the back of the ankle, the head, and the buttocks. The nodules don't usually occur early in the disease and are present in only about 30 percent of all patients.

Along with the tenderness, pain, and swelling in joints, most patients with RA experience persistent fatigue and a general malaise or sense of not feeling well. You may also have a low-grade fever.

THE CAUSE OF RA

In spite of extensive research, the exact cause of RA remains a mystery. What is it that triggers the immune system to attack a healthy body, and why does it choose to go after the synovial cells? Intense, ongoing research is trying to answer these questions, but no single culprit has emerged so far as a definitive cause.

What scientists do know is that certain factors appear to play a role in determining who gets the disease. We'll discuss each factor below.

Gender

About 70 percent of all people with RA are women, which suggests that hormones may play a role. The risk for developing RA may be higher in women who have never been pregnant and in women in the first year after they've given birth. Also, women who take oral contraceptives may be able to delay the onset of RA.

The onset and severity of RA may also be linked to gender. Women may get the disease at an earlier age and have more severe RA than men. In a study that looked at 844 patients who had had RA for less than twelve months, the average age of the women was

fifty-four, while the average age of the men was sixty. Among patients ages twenty to thirty, there were five times as many women as
men with RA. The numbers evened out in the sixty-to-seventy age
group. The men in the study were also more likely to go into remission. After two years, 40 percent of the men in the study were
in remission, compared with 28 percent of the women.

Genes

Although RA is not an inherited condition in the same way that
sickle-cell anemia is, genes can raise your odds for developing the
disease. The genetics of RA have come under intensive study in recent years, thanks to a joint project created in 1997 by the National
Institutes of Health and the Arthritis Foundation. The effort is
called the North American Rheumatoid Arthritis Consortium
(NARAC), and it involves researchers at twelve different research
centers who have recruited families with two or more siblings who
have RA to study the genetic implications of the disease.

Research from NARAC efforts has made some important advances in our understanding of the role of genetics in RA. For one,
scientists have confirmed a linkage between RA and a cluster of
genes involved in immune function called the human leukocyte
antigen (HLA) complex. Particular HLA genes may also predict
how severe the disease is and how well it will respond to treatment.
NARAC research has found that certain other genes may also be
involved, and that these genes may raise the risk for other autoimmune diseases such as Type 1 diabetes and lupus.

Scientists involved in NARAC have also discovered a specific
genetic variation that appears to double the risk for RA. The genetic
variation, called the single nucleotide polymorphism (SNP), is located in a gene that codes for an enzyme involved in controlling the
activation of T cells. SNP is found in about 28 percent of patients
with RA and about 17 percent of the general population. SNP was

also reported to be involved in the development of Type 1 diabetes and may be responsible for other autoimmune conditions, such as lupus and autoimmune thyroid disease.

But genes are only part of the equation. Not everyone who has these genes will develop RA. Studies have shown that when one person in a pair of identical twins has RA, the odds that the other twin will get the disease are only about one in three. Likewise, not everyone who has RA necessarily carries these genes. This lack of consistency in genetics makes the cause of RA even more difficult to determine.

Environment

Since gender and genes alone do not explain the development of RA, scientists suspect that other factors are involved in triggering the disease in people who are at risk. In fact, research suggests that the environment may play a bigger role than genetics. Although no single agent has been identified as an environmental cause of RA, several factors are possible, including:

- *Infection.* RA is not a contagious disease, but scientists have theorized that a virus or bacterium may be the culprit that causes RA in vulnerable people. But at this time, a viral or bacterial infection is strictly a theory, with no definitive evidence and no specific agent.
- *Hormones.* The fact that women are disproportionately affected by RA has prompted the hypothesis that hormones are somehow involved. For instance, women with RA tend to improve when they're pregnant, when the production of hormones increases substantially.
- *Cigarette smoking.* Although studies are inconclusive, most research suggests that smoking cigarettes raises your risk for developing RA. The risk appears to be related to the length

of time that you smoked and not how many cigarettes you smoked per day. Cigarette smoking may also increase the likelihood that your RA will be more severe.

- *Stress.* Whether it's physical trauma or emotional upheaval, scientists believe that anything that produces the stress response may play a role in the onset of RA. Some studies have suggested that major life events, such as divorce, death, and car accidents, are more frequent in the six months before the onset of RA.

- *Occupational hazards.* One recent study found that exposure to mineral dust and/or vibrations may increase your risk for developing RA. The study, which was conducted in Sweden, found that men who had been exposed to vibration, asphalt, asbestos, and organic and mineral dusts were more likely to develop RA. The study found that the chemicals were typically inhaled.

WHERE DOES IT GO FROM HERE?

Unfortunately, there is no cure for RA, and the course of this chronic disease is uncertain and unpredictable. For some people, the disease will eventually go into a remission, in which the pain lessens or disappears altogether and the joints become less swollen. During a remission, morning stiffness diminishes, and you may notice that you're no longer as tired as you've been and that your joints are no longer as painful, warm, or swollen.

In other patients, the symptoms may fluctuate for weeks or months. You may alternate between flare-ups, in which the disease is active and symptoms worsen, and remission. Often, this fluctuation is due to an adjustment to treatment, and the best patients become vigilant about taking good care of themselves and paying attention to their treatment so that they can help themselves as quickly as possible.

At its worst, RA may cause deformities of the hands and feet over time. The fingers may develop a condition known as ulnar deviation, in which the fingers bend toward the outer part of the arm, where the ulnar bone is located. Some patients experience "swan neck deformity," in which the middle joint of the finger bends down and the joint nearest the tip of the finger bends up, creating the appearance of a swan's neck. Patients may also develop boutonniere deformity, which occurs when the joint in the middle of a finger pops up. Some people may experience bowstring sign, in which the tendons on the back of the hand become prominent and taut.

Later on, as the disease progresses, there may be swelling in other larger joints such as the knees, hips, and cervical spine. In about 30 percent of people with RA, the disease causes inflammation of the cricoarytenoid joint, a joint near the windpipe, which can lead to hoarseness and difficulty breathing. Other organs and body parts that may become affected include:

- *The heart.* The tissue lining the chest cavity and surrounding the heart may become inflamed in a condition known as pericarditis and pericardial effusions. This condition causes chest pain and difficulty breathing.
- *The lungs.* Inflammation of the lining of the lungs causes pleurisy that may cause pleural effusions, leading to shortness of breath and a dry cough.
- *The nerves.* RA can cause a breakdown in the body's nervous system, which can lead to numbness, tingling, or weakness.
- *The eyes.* A condition known as scleritis, or inflammation of the whites of the eyes, may cause vision problems. RA is also linked to Sjögren's syndrome, a condition characterized by dry eyes and dry mouth. The dryness in the eyes can cause an irritating sensation, while dryness of the

mouth may make it difficult to chew or swallow. Women with Sjögren's syndrome may develop vaginal dryness.
- *The blood vessels.* With RA, some patients may experience inflammation of the blood vessels, or vasculitis.

Not everyone will develop these other conditions. And not everyone will experience a progressive worsening of the disease. But one thing is for sure: RA cannot go untreated and ignored. Over time, the disease can cause disabilities that could render you incapable of enjoying life.

WHAT DOES THE FUTURE HOLD FOR ME?

Fortunately, research has made great strides, and a diagnosis of RA is no longer as scary as it once was. Years ago, a patient with RA had little hope of escaping the long-term consequences of the disease and would most likely one day have to rely on a wheelchair.

It's true that RA can still take a major toll on your physical and emotional well-being. The disease can be very painful and may interfere with an individual's daily functioning, making it difficult to hold down a job, enjoy hobbies and activities, and care for loved ones. Having RA can also cause undue stress, depression, and anxiety. In addition, studies show that people who have RA are more likely to have other chronic conditions such as heart disease, lymphoma, and infections.

The goods news is that many of the symptoms can be effectively controlled and managed today. Early and aggressive treatment of the disease has made it possible for many people to avoid the consequences that once plagued those diagnosed with RA. New medications have proven to be extremely effective and in some cases have induced a full remission. Numerous patient support groups and self-management programs have also enabled patients to become more proactive in their own care. Proper self-care that involves making adjustments to your activity level, some lifestyle changes, and a balance of adequate rest and gentle exercise can help you achieve greater control of RA, too.

By reading this book, you are demonstrating your desire to learn more about this baffling disease and the treatment options and self-care measures that can help you manage it. That's good news for your health. According to the National Institute of Arthritis and Musculoskeletal and Skin Diseases, a branch of the National Institutes of Health, studies have shown that RA patients who are well-informed and actively participate in their own care have less pain and make fewer visits to the doctor than others with RA.

Learning as much as you can about RA will help you become familiar with the options available to you. It will also give you greater confidence and control over your condition. We hope that the information you glean from this book will help you live more effectively with RA.

PROFILE

MARCIA

All her life, Marcia had been healthy: She ate well, exercised, and maintained a healthy weight. So when the aches and pains of rheumatoid arthritis (RA) attacked her body, Marcia went into serious denial, thinking she could somehow correct her condition.

"I kept thinking, 'Oh, it'll go away, it'll go into remission,'" says Marcia, now fifty-one. "But I know now that if you have moderate to severe RA, it stays with you."

RA crept into her life shortly after she turned forty. A stabbing sensation in her right forearm, a soreness in the soles of her feet, and a general feeling of malaise made her aware that something was amiss. Then the pain began to attack her joints. "It was as if someone put a knife in my joints, then poured concrete into them," she says. The pain in her feet worsened, and it felt, she says, as if she were running barefoot over gravel.

Her family doctor put her on prednisone and referred her to a rheumatologist to confirm his suspicions. That's when she was diagnosed with RA and given Plaquenil. Marcia grew desperate, thinking for sure the diagnosis had been a mistake. She tried alternative remedies like eating golden raisins soaked in gin. She took fish oil supplements. She drank green tea. But her most rigorous effort to control the disease was to radically change her diet. She eliminated all sugar and fat from her diet and began eating only salad and taking supplements. She thought that if she ate only healthy foods, she'd be able to get her disease under control.

Her weight plummeted from a healthy 125 to 104. Her cholesterol dipped to 80 mg/DL. She was so weak she could barely move. Even brushing her teeth or going to the bathroom was a challenge. "I almost starved myself to death," she says. "But I kept thinking, 'This cannot be happening to me. It has to be something I'm eating. I'm going to heal myself. I do not have RA.'"

Instead, Marcia thought she might have Lyme disease. A few weeks before the aches and pain started, she had found a tick on her body. So she went to the Mayo Clinic, but they confirmed she had RA. "My husband told me that he'd take me to Mayo if I promised I'd accept the diagnosis and move forward with it, not backward," she says.

Then Marcia got another wake-up call: Her sister, a woman she called her best friend, was diagnosed with a malignant brain tumor. "It certainly put my illness in perspective," Marcia says. "Things were going to get worse, and I was going to have to get back on my feet to help her."

Marcia started taking higher doses of prednisone and experimenting with other medications that would eventually get her off the prednisone. She also began eating better and regaining the weight she had lost.

While taking care of her sister, Marcia continued to work in an optometrist's office, where she did book work, tended to patients, and did some accounting. As her RA worsened, it became increasingly difficult to work on eyewear. The RA made it hard to screw in lenses and to perform the fine motor tasks of assembling glasses. In 1995, after her son graduated from college, Marcia stopped working.

The following year, her father had heart surgery, her brother was in an accident, and her sister died. It was her unshakeable faith in God, she says, that got her through those dark days and helped her stay focused on her own healing.

As Marcia came to accept her own illness, she learned that nothing works for RA except rest, exercise, medications, and a positive attitude. Her medication regimen today includes methotrexate, Remicade, and Celebrex. She has also learned to take daily naps and to say no to the myriad volunteer opportunities at her church that come her way.

"I used to be on the run all day long," she says. "Nobody could outdo me. I could outrun anybody. Now I know that the world will go on if I'm not there all the time. I've found out that other people are just as capable as I am."

Instead of constantly being on the run, Marcia now focuses her energies on things that give her true pleasure and responsibilities that really matter. These include taking care of her father's house since her mother's death a year ago and pressing his shirts, tending her flowers, going to church, and taking walks with a good friend three or four times a week. She is also eagerly awaiting the arrival of her first grandchild.

CHAPTER TWO ✒

Making the Diagnosis

It's easy to dismiss the early symptoms of rheumatoid arthritis as something else, especially if the symptoms come on slowly. An achy finger might make you suspect long days at the computer. A swollen knee could be blamed on too much time spent in a tough spinning class. Fatigue is easily attributed to the rigors of your daily routine, so full of obligations to your job, your family, and your home.

Not surprisingly then, a diagnosis of RA does not come quickly or easily. There is no single test, sign, or symptom that reveals you have RA. To make diagnosis even more challenging, the disease presents itself differently in every patient. One patient might feel the first twinges of pain and experience swelling in her fingers. Another might feel it in her feet. Still a third might experience pain in her knees, shoulders, and hips. The challenge gets even more difficult when you consider that there are more than 100 different kinds of arthritis.

But a physician may begin to suspect RA if the pain is experienced symmetrically. That means if the joints of your right hand are experiencing pain and inflammation, you'll feel similar symptoms on the left side. Your physician may also suspect RA if the pain is especially pronounced in the mornings or after periods of inactivity, it's been around for six weeks or longer, and it is accompanied by stiffness, redness, and warmth. Other indications include fever, fatigue, and a general sense of malaise.

Getting to a diagnosis of RA doesn't happen in one single visit to the doctor. Chances are, he'll need to do blood tests, X-rays, and other procedures to get to the bottom of it.

THE OFFICIAL GUIDELINES

A diagnosis of RA is based on a physician's examination and observation, the patient's self-reported symptoms, blood tests, and X-rays. In 1987, the American College of Rheumatology (ACR) developed a seven-item list of criteria for a patient to be diagnosed with RA. A patient must have at least four of the seven criteria, and numbers one to four must have been present for at least six weeks. They are:

1. Morning stiffness in and around the joints, lasting at least one hour before maximal improvement.
2. Arthritis of three or more joint areas. At least three joint areas simultaneously have had soft tissue swelling (not bony overgrowth alone) or fluid observed by a physician. The fourteen possible areas are the right or left proximal interphalangeal (PIP) knuckle joints, the metacarpophalangeal (MCP) knuckle joints in the middle of the fingers, the wrist, elbow, knee, ankle, and the metatarsophalangeal (MTP) joints of the toes.
3. Arthritis of hand joints. At least one area swollen in a wrist, MCP, or PIP joint.
4. Symmetric arthritis. Simultaneous involvement of the same joint areas on both sides of the body.

5. Rheumatoid nodules. These free-floating lumps range in size from that of a millet grain to a golf ball and are visible to the physician. They're commonly found on the elbow, the back of the head, the sacrum (the last bone of the spine), the Achilles tendon, and the tendons of the hand. Although these nodules are strong indicators of RA, they occur in only 30 percent of patients with the disease.
6. Serum rheumatoid factor. Abnormal amounts of serum rheumatoid factor detected by a test that is positive in less than 5 percent of healthy people.
7. Radiographic changes. X-rays of the hand and wrist that show erosions or unequivocal bony decalcifications in or adjacent to the affected joints.

The ACR criteria can be helpful in making a diagnosis, though some doctors can detect RA even if a patient doesn't fully meet these guidelines. In fact, the ACR originally created the criteria to provide uniform research standards, allowing doctors and medical experts to do research, reports, and clinical studies among patients with comparable symptoms.

GETTING AN ANSWER

Trying to determine whether you have RA is a rigorous process that typically involves several visits to your doctor. Here are the various components of your visit that your doctor will use to get to a diagnosis of RA.

Medical History

Most physicians will begin by getting a thorough medical history from you. Possible questions might include: Where does it hurt? How long have you had these symptoms? When do they tend to occur? How have they affected your daily activities? Do you have a family history of arthritis or RA?

Physical Examination

Using a trained eye, your physician will closely observe your joints, looking for redness, warmth, and swelling. The swelling may indicate effusion, a buildup of excess fluid in your joints, or synovitis, inflammation of the joint lining. Your doctor will also check the range of motion in your joints and look for rheumatoid nodules and a loss of muscle mass. All are possible indicators of RA.

Besides closely examining your joints and muscles, your physician will take your blood pressure; check your glands; examine your eyes, ears, nose, and throat; and listen to your heart and lungs.

Blood Tests

If he suspects RA, your physician will order a series of blood tests. Certain markers in the blood are indicators for RA, but again, no single marker identifies a patient as having RA. Possible markers for RA include:

- **Rheumatoid factor (RF).** Approximately 70 to 80 percent of people with RA have rheumatoid factor in their blood. RF is an antibody produced by white blood cells. Although prevalent in RA patients, RF is also present in people with other inflammatory conditions as well as people who have no illness. And only 50 percent of people with RA will test positive for RF in the early stages of disease, which further limits its usefulness as a marker for RA.
- **Anti-CCP antibodies.** The measure of antibodies to cyclic citrulline-containing peptides has emerged as a new and improved way to detect RA. In fact, one study reported in the *Annals of Rheumatic Disease* found that the anti-CCP test was effective in identifying patients with RA more than 90 percent of the time, compared with the RF test, which was about 80 percent effective. Scientists believe the test

may predict the eventual development of RA in patients whose arthritis is undifferentiated and may even detect RA in healthy people years before the onset of disease.

- **Erythrocyte sedimentation rate (ESR).** The sed rate test, as it is also called, is one way to measure inflammation in the body. The test measures how quickly red blood cells settle in a test tube. In the presence of inflammation, certain proteins cause red blood cells, or erythrocytes, to settle faster, resulting in a higher ESR. Though the ESR is useful for gauging the presence of inflammation and the effectiveness of treatment, it is not sufficient by itself for diagnosing RA because elevated levels are present in other inflammatory conditions, such as infection.
- **C-reactive protein (CRP).** Like the ESR, the CRP test is a gauge of inflammation. These proteins are produced in the liver and rise in the presence of inflammatory conditions. But like the ESR, this test alone is not indicative of RA.
- **Antinuclear antibodies (ANA).** People who have connective tissue diseases often produce this antibody, but ANAs are sometimes also present in healthy people. Testing for antinuclear antibodies may also help differentiate other conditions such as lupus, scleroderma, Sjögren's syndrome, and mixed connective tissue disease.

In rare cases, the doctor may also test for genetic markers when ordering blood work. More specifically, he will look for two genetic markers:

- **HLA-DR4 and DR-1.** These genetic markers can be found on the surface of specific white blood cells. Approximately two-thirds of Caucasians with RA have these

genetic markers, and their presence may indicate susceptibility for RA. At the same time, however, many people
who have these markers do not have RA, making these
markers inconclusive tools for diagnosis.

- **HLA-B27.** People who suffer from a form of inflammatory
  arthritis such as ankylosing spondylitis and reactive arthritis
  often carry this genetic marker. This genetic marker is often
  more a tool for ruling out other diseases.

People who have RA may also have other blood abnormalities,
including anemia, which is a reduction in red blood cells; leukocytosis, an overproduction of white blood cells; and thrombocytosis,
excessive production of platelets, the substance responsible for clotting. But all of these abnormalities can occur in other conditions
and are not specific to RA.

Imaging Studies

Patient reports, observations, and blood work are sometimes still not
enough for a diagnosis, so your physician may use X-rays to determine whether you have RA. But sometimes the damage to your bones
cannot be seen early on. Erosions, which resemble tiny holes in the
bone, typically appear on the MCP and PIP joints of the hands, for
instance, and can be identified on X-rays in only 15 to 30 percent of
patients in the first year of disease. After the first two years, those erosions can be seen in approximately 90 percent of the patients.

Your doctor may also use X-rays to look for thinning of the
bone in the areas near the joints as well as a shrinkage of joint
space between the bones, which indicates a loss of joint cartilage.

Other imaging techniques that your doctor may use include:

- **Magnetic resonance imaging (MRI).** Using a magnet
  to create vibrations in a targeted area, the MRI produces a

detailed image on a computer. MRIs are considerably more sensitive than X-rays, but also more costly. For one, the MRI can detect bone erosions earlier in the disease than an X-ray can. When X-rays and MRIs were compared in a group of patients with early arthritis, the MRI identified seven times more erosions in the MCP and PIP joints than the plain radiographs. MRIs are also able to detect the abnormal growth of synovial tissue.

- **Computerized axial tomography (CAT or CT scans).** These advanced X-rays shoot several X-rays from different vantage points, which are then viewed on a computer screen, not film. Both CAT scans and MRIs are more sophisticated than X-rays and can reveal information about tissues such as muscle, cartilage, and joints.

Other Diagnostic Tools

Sometimes, making the diagnosis may be particularly challenging, and your doctor may need to perform additional procedures to confirm that you have RA. Possible tools he might use include:

- **Arthrocentesis.** In this procedure, the rheumatologist uses a needle and inserts it into the joint to remove fluid for examination. The fluid will reveal the amount of inflammation in the joint and can help exclude other conditions such as gout and infection.
- **Ultrasound.** Studies show that advances in technology have made ultrasound a potentially viable tool in the diagnosis of RA. The technique provides visual images of inflammation and damage in the small joints of the hands and feet.
- **Needle biopsy.** Using a needle, the doctor removes a small piece of the synovium, or joint lining, for examination. This procedure is rarely done for diagnosis and is

more often a research tool to determine the effectiveness of medications. It can also help rule out unusual infections such as tuberculosis.

- **Arthroscopy.** This procedure uses a tool called an arthroscope to look into the joint through an incision in the skin. An arthroscope is a very thin tube with a light at the end. On the other end, it is connected to a closed-circuit television that allows the physician to see the extent of joint damage. Arthroscopy is more often used as a therapeutic intervention than as a diagnostic tool.

WHAT RA IS NOT

Getting to a diagnosis of RA is not easy. Many of the symptoms overlap with other conditions, and it may be difficult for the doctor to determine exactly what you have. Below are some conditions that may be mistaken for RA.

Osteoarthritis

Osteoarthritis (OA), also called degenerative joint disease, is one of the most common types of arthritis and afflicts about sixteen million people. The disease is characterized by the breakdown of the cartilage inside the joint, which causes the bones to rub together. Cartilage, as you may recall, is the cushioning at the ends of the bones. The result is pain and a decrease in the range of motion. Common joints affected include those at the end of the fingers and the bottom of the thumb, the knees, hips, and those in the feet and back.

OA runs the range from very mild to extremely severe. It typically affects people as they age, though the condition is not an inevitable condition of age, nor is it limited to older people. Injuries from sports or work-related activities as well as obesity can raise your risk for developing OA. People who are born with defective cartilage or with slight defects in the joints are also prone to OA.

Systemic Lupus Erythematosus

Often called the great imitator, systemic lupus erythematosus (SLE), or lupus, is a difficult to diagnose disease whose symptoms mimic those of other conditions. Like RA, lupus is an autoimmune condition in which the body's immune system turns on its own healthy tissues. In lupus, the damage can occur in multiple parts of the body, including the joints, skin, kidneys, heart, lungs, blood vessels, and brain. Approximately 500,000 to a million people in the United States have lupus.

Symptoms of the disease range from mild to severe and include painful or swollen joints, fatigue, unexplained fever, skin rashes, and kidney problems. Patients often develop a rash on the face and may experience hair loss, sensitivity to the sun, and extreme sensitivity in the fingers or toes in reaction to cold and stress. Patients typically fluctuate between flare-ups and periods of remission.

Fibromyalgia

Like lupus, fibromyalgia is difficult to diagnose because its symptoms resemble those of other conditions. People who have fibromyalgia endure widespread musculoskeletal pain, fatigue, and tenderness in specific parts of their bodies, including the neck, spine, shoulders, and hips. The pain is intense and deep and may also be accompanied by numbness and tingling. People who have fibromyalgia may also suffer from severe sleep disturbances, migraine headaches, and irritable bowel syndrome. Experts estimate that the condition affects three to six million people in the United States.

Juvenile Rheumatoid Arthritis

Although it shares a similar name with RA, juvenile rheumatoid arthritis (JRA) is actually a different disease. As the name suggests, JRA usually affects children under the age of sixteen. Approximately 71,000 children in the United States have this condition, which is characterized by joint inflammation as well as pain, swelling, and stiffness. Because of the pain, some children will hold a sore joint in one particular position, which over time can result in stiff and weakened muscles. Long-lasting cases of JRA can result in joint damage and altered growth of the bones.

Gout

Unlike most other rheumatic diseases, gout is more common in men than in women. This painful condition results from a buildup of needle-shaped crystals of uric acid, a substance naturally produced by the body that is also a by-product produced by the breakdown of certain foods. The excess uric acid then settles in connective tissue, the joint space between bones, or both. The deposits create the symptoms of arthritis, namely swelling, redness, heat, pain, and joint stiffness. Gout is characterized by sporadic episodes of inflammation.

Spondyloarthropathies

There are five different diseases in this category: ankylosing spondylitis, Reiter's syndrome, psoriatic arthritis, arthritis/spondylitis associated with inflammatory bowel disease, and undifferentiated spondyloarthropathy. Three of them have symptoms that may be confused with RA:

- **Ankylosing spondylitis** typically begins in young adults in their twenties and thirties and is marked early on by pain and stiffness in the lower back and buttocks. Over time, the pain may spread upward and even to the neck. Some patients also develop arthritis in the arms and legs, and iritis or uveitis, inflammations of the eye.
- **Reactive arthritis,** which is sometimes called Reiter's syndrome, usually affects the joints of the knees, ankles, and

toes, and occasionally those in the hands and arms. Patients may also develop a rash on their hands or the soles of their feet. The condition may also be accompanied by inflammation of the eye.

- **Psoriatic arthritis** is a joint condition that can be seen in people with psoriasis, a skin condition that is characterized by a scaly rash that occurs on the scalp, elbows, knees, and/or the lower end of the spine. Some patients also develop nail lesions. The skin disease may precede the arthritis by a number of years, or the arthritis may come before the skin disease. In some cases, they may occur simultaneously.

Arthritis/spondylitis associated with inflammatory bowel disease is diagnosed when a patient has arthritis or inflammation in the joints along with Crohn's disease or ulcerative colitis. Crohn's disease involves inflammation of the colon or small intestines, and ulcerative colitis is characterized by ulcers and inflammation of the lining of the colon. The more severe the inflammatory bowel disease, the more severe the arthritis symptoms.

Undifferentiated spondyloarthropathy is usually diagnosed when the patient has a mix of signs and symptoms that don't seem to fit in just one category.

AN IMITATOR

Parvo B19 virus is a viral disease that can mimic RA. In young children, the virus presents itself as fifth disease, which appears as a rash and fever. Adults who don't have this disease in childhood may develop it later in a condition that resembles RA. Patients will experience pain and swelling in the joints, morning stiffness, and fatigue. The condition may last a couple of weeks or as long as up to two months, but it will then go away by itself. Unlike other conditions we have discussed, it is contagious.

A FINAL NOTE

Determining whether you have RA takes patience and perseverance. But once you get to a diagnosis, you'll be able to start working on finding the best treatment for your condition. You'll also be able to begin making the lifestyle modifications you need to get the disease under control. And that will help you achieve the relief you're seeking.

PROFILE

ELAINE

Most people who develop rheumatoid arthritis are diagnosed by a rheumatologist. For Elaine, it was an observant podiatrist who detected her RA.

Back in 1999, Elaine was taking step aerobics when the ball of her foot swelled up one night. "I thought I'd just landed on it wrong, so I went to see my doctor, who referred me to a podiatrist," she says.

Pain relievers prescribed by the podiatrist barely helped, so Elaine went back to the podiatrist's office. He took an X-ray and did some blood work. That's when he discovered she had RA and referred her to a rheumatologist.

Aches and pains were nothing new to Elaine, now fifty-two. She always attributed them to her job as a pre-K teacher or the rigors of toting her own three children around.

Finding the right medication regimen didn't come easily. Different medicines caused different side effects. Vioxx caused severe diarrhea. Plaquenil gave her terrible stomach pains and aggravated her irritable bowel syndrome. Methotrexate made her nauseous and eventually stopped working. Twice a month, she gave herself painful injections of Humira, and she eventually tired of giving herself weekly shots of Enbrel.

Equally distressing were the overwhelming fatigue and her increasing inability to maintain a busy life. "I would come home from work and go right to bed," she says. "I had to drastically decrease my activity."

For Elaine, that meant giving up on her involvement with the town's Democratic committee and activities at her church, her children's schools, the local fire department, and the teacher's union at her job. She began missing meetings and stopped participating in events. "It took me two years to realize that I couldn't do all these things," she says. "That's when I got depressed. I got so discouraged and felt so depressed because I just couldn't keep up with myself. Everything I did was a major effort. When I got home, I couldn't function. My husband was doing all the laundry, and I had to hire someone to clean my house."

Elaine's doctor put her on an antidepressant, and she sought counseling. But even so, she wondered whether her depression was really the result of menopause. "It was my doctor who told me that this depression was all part of the disease," she says.

Eventually, Elaine found a drug that helped tame her RA: Remicade. For the last two years, she's been going to her doctor's office every four to five weeks and sitting for a two- to three-hour intravenous infusion of Remicade. She's also been in remission for more than a year.

Over the years, Elaine has learned that certain things can affect her RA. Stress and fatigue can trigger a flare-up, as can eating too many tomatoes or tomato sauce. Carrying heavy grocery bags also can create pain.

On the other hand, eating more high-protein foods, such as chicken, eggs, tuna, or almonds, seems to provide relief. And to ensure a good night's sleep, Elaine sometimes takes Aventyl.

Although she has adjusted to her slower pace, Elaine still has days when she misses doing all that she used to do, especially her crafts. She used to sew quilts by hand but now does them by machine. She also used to do stenciling and candlewicking but has given them up.

Elaine would also love to try her hand at gardening, but she doesn't want to start anything she can't finish. "I want to do these hobbies, but I don't have the energy anymore," she says.

What she has found the energy for is spending time with her family, taking walks with her husband whenever she can, and staying on top of her medical condition. She also continues working and has come to terms with her limitations. "It isn't always easy doing less than what I'd like to do," Elaine says. "But I've learned that it's the best thing I can do for myself."

CHAPTER THREE 🙠

Assembling a Medical Team

Having a disease like RA—or any rheumatic disease, for that matter—is undoubtedly challenging. The disease is unpredictable, chronic, and painful, and the symptoms are diverse and vary from one patient to the next. Finding the right treatment typically takes a great deal of trial and error. The frustration and emotional toil can be exhausting.

That's why it's so important that once you learn you have RA, you start putting together a good team of doctors to help with your care. Because the disease affects so many aspects of your life, RA often involves input from several health professionals. A rheumatologist is critical to monitoring your disease and making sure you take the right combination of medications. An occupational therapist may need to step in if you need help finding pain relief and assistance in performing day-to-day tasks. A social worker or psychologist may need to help you adjust to the emotional aspects of your disease.

Assembling your medical team is just a part of the process of managing your disease. Once you have pulled together a satisfactory team, you need to think of yourself as the person in charge and become thoroughly involved in your own care. You are the one who will determine the goals of your treatment, communicate among the team members, and provide the feedback they need to do their best. You should also keep track of all the medical information that's bandied about, including dates of medical appointments, lab test and X-ray results, and the various treatment regimens you try. In addition, you need to stay on top of developments in the study and treatment of RA, so that you can discuss them with your health-care providers.

All of this medical management, record-keeping, and education may seem overwhelming at first. But studies show that patient education and involvement is critical to how well the disease is controlled and managed. The more involved and better educated you are, the better your prognosis.

That's why it's so important to put together a team of health-care professionals that is competent in managing RA. You should feel comfortable discussing your health with these critical players and have confidence in their judgment and capabilities.

THE MEMBERS OF YOUR MEDICAL TEAM
When choosing your team, think of yourself as the captain of a sports team. You want to choose the best players for each position, so when each one does his job, the whole team benefits. Let's take a look at the medical team you need to aid in your care.

General Practitioner or Family Physician
Back before you were diagnosed, you probably saw no other doctor except your general practitioner (GP) or family physician. In fact, early appointments to discuss your arthritis pain may even have begun with your GP. Chances are, your GP was the one who referred you to a rheumatologist.

While you probably won't see your family physician for your RA, you may still see him for minor ailments unrelated to your RA.

When it comes to treating RA, you will definitely need a skilled rheumatologist, although your family physician should be kept informed about the treatment you are receiving for your RA.

Rheumatologist

Because diagnosing and treating RA can be so challenging, it's important that you have a good rheumatologist on board. An astute rheumatologist is especially important to your medical team because early, aggressive treatment of RA ultimately improves the control and management of the disease.

Rheumatologists specialize in the diagnosis and treatment of arthritis, certain autoimmune disorders, conditions involving musculoskeletal pain, and osteoporosis. Becoming a rheumatologist requires extensive training.

After four years of medical school and three years of training in internal medicine, rheumatologists spend another two to three years in rheumatology training. Most choose to become board certified, which requires passing a rigorous exam conducted by the American Board of Internal Medicine.

While in training, rheumatologists learn the skills it takes to determine whether a patient has RA or another kind of auto-immune disease or arthritis. They learn to read X-rays of joints and to understand the ways different medications work in the body. But a skilled rheumatologist doesn't end his training with medical school or board certification. A good rheumatologist should be on top of all the latest research and developments in the diagnosis and treatment of RA.

So how do you know if a particular rheumatologist is the right one for you? That will depend on individual preference. A doctor's office location could be important to you, if you have difficulty traveling long distances. Or maybe it's important to you to have a physician who communicates without using medical lingo. Perhaps you're willing to tolerate a doctor with a poor bedside manner in exchange for superior technical competence.

Here are some good questions to answer to help you determine whether a doctor is right for you:

- Does the rheumatologist specialize in the treatment of RA? Does he already have many patients with RA? A rheumatologist who has dealt with many other RA patients is generally more skilled at identifying symptoms and prescribing appropriate treatments. And that means he will be better equipped to treat your unique case.
- What kinds of alliances does the rheumatologist have with other health-care professionals? Does she have other people in her practice who can assist in your care? Is she plugged in to a network of other medical professionals or affiliated with a good hospital?
- What kinds of health insurance does the rheumatologist accept?
- What kind of communication skills does the rheumatologist have? Do you feel comfortable in his presence? Does he listen to what you say and ask for your input and ideas? Does he answer your questions in words that you understand? Does he call you back when you need assistance or information?
- How convenient is the office to your home or work place? Are appointments easy to get? Does the staff treat you well?

Advanced Practice Nurse

Registered nurses who go on to meet advanced educational and clinical practice requirements also play a role in the treatment of patients with RA. These nurses work with patients and their families to help develop a plan of care. They may also prescribe, order, and implement treatments, assist in counseling for the patient and her family, and initiate referrals to other health-care providers.

Physical Therapist

Patients who are suffering from extreme pain or need help with physical recovery may turn to a physical therapist (PT) for assistance. PTs work to bolster a patient's independence and self-sufficiency by developing a physical treatment plan that addresses his or her pain.

The PT may use numerous techniques to reduce your pain, including exercise, hydrotherapy, electrical stimulation, heat, and cold. After getting an assessment and doing a physical exam, the PT will work with you to devise a program of rest and exercise that improves your function. By devising exercises that strengthen your muscles, improve your range of motion, and bolster your cardiovascular conditioning, your PT can help restore some of your vitality.

Occupational Therapist

Buttoning a shirt. Tying your shoes. Climbing into your car. We take these mundane activities for granted when we're healthy. But even the most simple of tasks in your daily routine can become a monumental challenge when you're encumbered by the pain of RA. Inflamed joints are also at greater risk for injury than healthy joints.

That's where an occupational therapist (OT) can help. Think of the OT as the most practical player on your team, the one who will teach you how to move through your daily routine in ways that cause less pain and that put your joints at less risk. The OT also helps you find ways to conserve energy, so that you never overexert yourself. In addition, an OT can help you find the splints and equipment you need to protect your joints, reduce your pain, and improve your function.

Ophthalmologist

Having RA and taking the medications you need for it often puts your eyes at risk for problems. Some people with RA experience dryness in the eyes and mouth, a condition known as sicca syndrome. About 1 percent of RA patients will develop scleritis, a chronic inflammation of the blood vessels in the whites of the eyes that produces pain and redness.

People with RA are also at increased risk for secondary Sjögren's syndrome, a chronic condition that occurs when the body's immune system mistakenly attacks moisture-producing glands, including the tear glands, causing eyes to have a gritty feeling and burning sensation. Other eye conditions associated with RA are uveitis, inflammation of the uveal tract of the eye, and iritis, inflammation of the iris.

Certain medications you take for RA can also produce problems. Patients taking hydroxychloroquine (Plaquenil), for instance, need to have periodic evaluations with an ophthalmologist to monitor damage to the retina. And prednisone, a steroid, can worsen cataracts or cause glaucoma. Irritations of the eye require the attention of an ophthalmologist, a medical doctor trained to treat these conditions.

Social Worker

Patients who need community support or resources may often turn to a social worker for assistance. Social workers get involved in the psychosocial aspects of the patient's life by offering counseling, seeking out services in the community that can assist a patient in her return to independence, and helping to identify resources that can address a patient's need for financial help, home care, transportation, and support groups.

Pharmacist

Medications play a critical role in the management of RA. But given the costly medications involved in treating RA, it may be more likely that you'll be getting your medications from a mail-order pharmacy (see chapter seven), which is fine.

If you're fortunate enough, you may develop a personal relationship with a pharmacist. In that case, it's best to choose a pharmacist you like and trust, and to then use that person for all your prescriptions. By sticking with one pharmacist, you'll have someone who keeps a comprehensive file of all the drugs you are taking. If you use a pharmacist only on occasion—to obtain that once-in-a-while antibiotic or cough remedy—make sure that person knows all the RA medications you take.

But don't view your pharmacist solely as a person who dispenses medications. Pharmacists are a wealth of information. They can alert you to potentially dangerous drug interactions and possible side effects from any medications you're prescribed. Pharmacists can tell you whether an over-the-counter remedy will interact with a prescription medication you're taking. Plus, they can advise you on whether drugs require food before they're ingested.

Psychologist

Having RA means more than just adapting to arthritis pain and fatigue. The disease also takes a tremendous emotional toll. Living with a chronic illness that is potentially disabling can cause a constellation of emotional and psychological symptoms such as anger, depression, fear, and anxiety. Patients may also experience difficulties in their personal relationships, work situations, and families.

A psychologist can help you work through these myriad issues through counseling and therapy. After a thorough discussion and evaluation of your problems, a psychologist can help you devise the coping skills you need to overcome these difficulties. He or she can also teach you mind-body techniques that enhance relaxation and bolster your pain management.

Other People You Might Need

The health-care professionals we've discussed so far are the leading members of your team, the health professionals you're most likely to need. But because RA varies so much from one patient to the next, you may need some other medical professionals to come on board from time to time. These people include:

- **Orthopedic surgeon.** These doctors evaluate and treat disorders and diseases of the bones, joints, tendons, and ligaments. They may perform arthroscopy to peer inside your joints in order to determine the source of your problems or to do a biopsy of the inflamed tissue. Orthopedic surgeons also perform surgical procedures, including those on the shoulders, elbows, hips, and knees.
- **Podiatrist.** Many people who have RA suffer from foot problems such as swelling, stiffness, and pain. Eventually, you may experience deformities in your feet, which make it difficult to walk and to find shoes that fit well. A podiatrist can help you treat some of these foot problems and also fit you for orthotics and custom-made shoes.
- **Registered dietitian (RD).** Although there is no special diet to alleviate the pain of RA, all people with chronic illnesses should pay close attention to what they eat. Excess weight can aggravate the symptoms of RA and worsen pressure on the joints. But certain medications you take for RA can make weight loss, even maintenance, difficult. Corticosteroids, for instance, stimulate the appetite. RA also causes the loss of muscle, which can lower your metabolic rate, again causing weight gain. A registered dietitian can help you learn how to eat more nutritiously and in ways that will help limit weight gain.

KEEPING GOOD MEDICAL RECORDS

Now that you've assembled a good medical team that has your complete confidence, you might think you're free to let them keep track of your care. Unfortunately, that's not true. As part of your continued involvement, you will need to keep track of all the information. Think of yourself as the central clearinghouse for all of your medical information.

Doctors make a lot of medical decisions based on what you tell them. That's why it's important that you know what other healthcare professionals have told you. Here is some important information that you should keep track of:

- **Your medical visits.** Use a journal to jot down the dates of all of your visits, including dental checkups. Record the purpose of your visit, symptoms, and any medications you were prescribed. Also record your height, weight, and blood pressure.
- **Consultation reports from specialists.** If you see a specialist, ask him to share his report of the visit with you. These narrative reports provide comprehensive descriptions of your symptoms, the exam, and any lab findings. They also offer an analysis of the problem and a plan of action.
- **Lab tests.** Get copies of all blood test results and X-rays. If necessary, give the receptionist a self-addressed, stamped envelope to ensure you get the information.
- **Preventive screenings.** Even if the findings show you're healthy, it's important to keep a record of the results.
- **Discharge summaries for overnight hospitalizations.** The summaries are written by your physician and discuss the procedures you underwent, the diagnosis, and the status

of your health during your stay. If you have an outpatient procedure, ask for an operative report, which details your visit.

AFFORDING THE TEAM

Let's face it: Having RA isn't cheap. Between the multiple doctor visits, the prescription medications, and the visits to specialists, the cost of RA can be quite high. Experts estimate that RA costs approximately five billion dollars a year, with the bulk of those costs attributed to hospitalizations and home nursing care. And if you become disabled from having RA, you may lose the income you need to afford your care.

But getting the proper care you need is critical to your health and well-being. According to the Arthritis Foundation, good medical coverage is one of the most important assets you can have when you develop a chronic condition like RA. When looking for a group or individual policy, the foundation suggests checking for:

- **Outpatient and inpatient care.** Check that the policy covers doctor visits as well as outpatient services, surgery, and hospital care. The plan should cover surgeries that relieve pain and promote function.
- **Doctor choice.** Some insurance policies, such as those offered by a Health Maintenance Organization (HMO) or Preferred Provider Organization (PPO), limit the healthcare professionals you can see. Is your rheumatologist a participating provider in the plan's network? Are there enough specialists in your plan?
- **Rehabilitation coverage.** A good insurance plan should cover the cost of occupational, physical, and vocational therapy. It should also cover assisting devices such as walkers, braces, splints, and computer-assistance devices.

- **Prescription drug coverage.** Make sure the insurance plan provides coverage for prescription drugs. Ask to see the plan's formulary, which lists the drugs the plan will cover. Medications for RA are typically very expensive and require prior authorization.
- **Laboratory and other monitoring procedures.** Check that the plan covers lab tests that not only diagnose a condition but also monitor the impact of medications and therapies.
- **Costs.** What kind of costs will you incur from your plan? What are the premiums, deductibles, and co-payments?
- **Service.** Call the insurer's customer service phone number and see how quickly you get help.
- **Health plan report card.** Some insurance plans get rated by consumer groups for customer satisfaction and quality of care. Check to see if such a rating exists for a plan you're considering.

A FINAL NOTE

Once you have your team together, remember one thing: You are in charge. It's up to you to schedule the appointments, seek answers, and keep records. No one doctor will have every shred of information regarding your condition—only you will have that. Work with your medical team to get the best care possible. That means communicating your concerns at every turn. Nothing is more important than taking care of your health.

PROFILE

MARGARET

While most people experience early symptoms of RA in their joints, Margaret's first symptoms appeared in her eyes.

Back in 1983, while working at a college library, Margaret came down with sudden excruciating pain in her eye. The next day, her eye was flaming red and unbearably painful. She went to see an ophthalmologist, who told her she had iritis, an inflammation of the iris of the eye. Bright lights stung her eyes, and her whites remained bloodshot.

Eventually, she was also diagnosed with uveitis, an inflammation of the uvea of the eye. Her doctor prescribed prednisone drops, which she used every hour. The prednisone caused the pressure to build up in her eye, and Margaret wound up with glaucoma.

Although it took many years, Margaret began to notice that her eye problems always seemed to coincide with pain in her joints. At a visit to her ophthalmologist's office in 1999, she heard him mention the words *flare-up*. "That's when it connected," says Margaret, sixty, who now works as a librarian at a newspaper. "Could the pain in my joints be connected to what was happening in my eyes? I mentioned it to the doctor, but he didn't say much, and I didn't push it."

Then, on September 22, 1999—Margaret remembers the exact date—she awoke to find she was totally immobile. "Every part of my body was in pain," she recalls. "I couldn't get out of bed. I fell onto my knees and pulled myself up using the bed. My ankles and feet hurt and were terribly swollen."

She immediately called her doctor, who said she had arthritis and needed to get to a rheumatologist right away. A blood test suggested she had lupus, but the rheumatologist was skeptical. "I didn't have the rash, and I didn't have any sores in my mouth," Margaret says. "I just didn't have enough symptoms of lupus."

In January 2000, Margaret was finally told she had RA. She was immediately put on methotrexate. The pain gradually worsened. She had times when her feet were so swollen she could wear nothing but sandals simply because she couldn't get her shoes on. She also had aches in her wrists and knuckles.

In spite of it all, Margaret never missed a day of work. Few people even knew she was sick. One person she did tell was her boss, who helped re-arrange her working space to make it more comfortable and user-friendly.

Still, getting through a day wasn't easy. "It took me an hour and a half to get dressed every single day, and it took me half an hour to get my shoes on," she says. "Some days, I'd get to work, and I could barely move. There were days when I'd just sit at my desk and cry my eyes out. Sometimes after work, I'd get in my car and just bawl and cry because it just hurt so much. I could really see myself in a wheelchair."

About a year after she started taking methotrexate, she started feeling bet-ter. In the fall of 2003, Margaret went into remission. But she continues to take methotrexate to help keep the disease under control and to help tame the flare-ups from her iritis.

The drug has caused her to lose her hair, and she now wears a wig. She's also developed a rheumatoid nodule on her right hand. The bottom part of her left thumb sticks up in the air. But the changes in physical appearance are bear-able now that the pain has let up. "I just feel so lucky I'm walking," she says.

CHAPTER FOUR ❧

Living with RA

The French impressionist painter Pierre-Auguste Renoir had rheumatoid arthritis and tied a paintbrush to his hand in order to continue painting. Actress Lucille Ball had it as a teenager and wore orthopedic braces for years, before going on to become one of the most beloved comediennes in Hollywood history. Christiaan Barnard was bothered by RA much of his life, but became the first surgeon in the world to perform a heart transplant in 1967.

Clearly, RA does not have to get in the way of your dreams and goals.

But that doesn't mean that having RA won't have an impact on your daily life. You already know you'll be at more doctor's appointments and following a strict regimen of medications. But what kind of a toll will RA have on the rest of your life? How will it affect your energy levels? Your ability to hold down a job? Your hobby of traveling? In this chapter, we'll discuss the day-to-day challenges of living with this chronic illness. Keep in mind that because the disease varies so much from one patient to the next, you may experience symptoms that are better or worse than someone else.

LIVING WITH CHRONIC PAIN

If you're like most people, you probably took for granted how easy it was to use a can opener, turn a doorknob, or climb into a car. Now that you have RA, these simple everyday motions may be more challenging as you battle the pain of the disease.

What exactly is pain? Pain is a sensation detected in nerve endings, which is then transmitted to our brains. It is a signal that alerts you to the fact that something is wrong in your body, be it your fingertip coming into contact with a hot stove, your elbow striking a doorway, or a pounding headache brought on by the stress of your morning commute. In patients with RA, pain is a defense mechanism, your body's way of protecting itself against the damage that is taking place in your joints. Unlike pain that occurs with an injury—which is acute, short-term, and goes away as the injury heals—the pain you have from RA is chronic, which means it may fluctuate but will usually last a lifetime.

The pain of RA is caused by several factors, including inflammation, joint tissue damage, fatigue, depression, and stress. Swelling within the joint can bring on pain, as can the simple act of climbing out of bed in the morning. Every person has a different threshold for pain, which is affected not only by your physical tolerance for pain but also by your emotional and mental states.

Minimizing the pain is critical to your quality of life. Through a combination of medications, rest, exercise, and other therapies, you can reduce the amount of pain you're experiencing. Establishing the proper mix, however, can take a lot of trial and error, which requires a lot of patience.

In your battle against pain, it's also important to devote time to being with friends and family, to keep a positive attitude, and to maintain a sense of humor. Continuing to do the activities you enjoyed before you got sick can minimize your pain as well. So if you enjoy helping others, consider doing volunteer work in your community or church. If you always liked traveling, make sure to find time to get away. If you like gardening, try to find ways to continue your hobby. When you do these activities, realize that you may have to scale back a bit. For instance, if you always enjoyed long hikes on vacation, you may have to take shorter walks now.

Relaxation techniques, massage, and hot or cold packs can reduce your pain, too. In addition, it's important to get enough sleep, eat a balanced diet, and get some exercise. Taking care of your overall health and well-being can go a long way toward reducing your pain.

COPING WITH CHRONIC FATIGUE

Having RA often means experiencing overwhelming feelings of fatigue. One woman likened it to the first trimester of pregnancy, but compounded by the persistent pain in her joints. And for some patients, the challenges of living with chronic fatigue are as bad as, if not worse than, living with chronic pain.

The source of your fatigue can be complicated. Some patients are tired because the pain of RA is preventing them from getting a good night's sleep. The lack of a good night's sleep can exacerbate the pain. But other factors might also be involved:

- People who have RA are also vulnerable to anemia, low levels of red blood cells, which reduces the amount of hemoglobin in your blood and therefore the amount of oxygen circulating in your cells.
- Having a disease like RA can hamper your levels of physical activity. Like lack of sleep, inactivity can create a cycle of fatigue. Arthritis pain makes it hard for you to exercise, which causes you to lose overall conditioning and muscle strength. The resulting fatigue makes it even harder for you to exercise, which worsens the fatigue.

- A debilitating illness like RA can cause depression in even the most optimistic people. Being depressed on a regular basis can often cause fatigue.
- Eating well is difficult for people who have RA. Chronic pain may dampen your appetite, and if the pain is in your hands or wrists, you might find it difficult to prepare a healthy meal. A bad diet can cause fatigue.

The Importance of Sleep

For patients with RA, sleep becomes critical. Gone are the days when you burned the candle at both ends, stayed up late to watch a favorite TV show, or juggled numerous responsibilities simply for the thrill of it. As a person living with RA, it's important that you make a serious effort to get a good night's rest every single night. A good night's sleep not only combats fatigue but also helps you cope with the pain, boosts your energy, and improves your mood. Lack of sleep, or frequent insomnia, can cause depression.

Sometimes, though, the pain of RA can affect your sleep habits, making it difficult for you to get the rest you need. To overcome sleep difficulties, start by improving your sleep habits. Consider some of the following strategies:

- Limit the amount of time you spend in bed.
- Do not use the bedroom for anything except sleep and sex. Move the television out of the room, and do your nighttime reading in another room. Avoid working in bed.
- If you can't sleep after fifteen minutes, get up and do something relaxing like reading or folding laundry. Then try again. If you still can't sleep, get up and do another mundane task before trying again.
- Avoid daytime naps. Napping during the day typically disrupts a good night's sleep.

- Do not eat or drink anything in the two hours before bed.
- Exercise regularly, but don't do it in the three hours before bedtime.
- Avoid alcohol and nicotine an hour or two before going to bed. (Ideally, eliminate both from your routine since both alcohol and nicotine are disruptive to a good night's rest.)
- Limit caffeine or ban it from your diet, especially later in the day.
- Go to bed and get up at the same time every day.
- Set aside a time just for worrying. If necessary, write your worries down in a notebook, then close it until morning.
- Create a relaxing bedtime ritual like a warm bath or listening to music that will help you get in the mood for sleep.

Medications for Insomnia

If sleep problems persist, you may need more than behavioral changes. Talk to your doctor, who may prescribe a sleep remedy. Prescription sleep medications include:

- Benzodiazepines, which include extazolam (ProSom), flurazepam (Dalmane), and temazepam (Restoril).
- Non-benzodiazepines, which include zolpidem (Ambien) and zaleplon (Sonata).
- Antidepressants, which include amitriptyline (Elavil), nortriptyline (Pamelor), nefazodone (Serzone), and trazodone (Desyrel).

You may also consider trying an over-the-counter (OTC) sleep medication. Many OTC remedies contain an antihistamine that causes a sedating effect. Alternately, you may consider using an herbal remedy. Two herbal remedies that have been found to promote sleep are valerian, a root that can be steeped in hot water for tea, and melatonin, a substance naturally produced by the body.

All medications for sleep need to be taken with care. Some can cause daytime drowsiness that lasts well into the next day. And people who drink alcohol should not take sleep medications since the combination intensifies the effects of both. These drugs should also not be used by people with breathing difficulties, glaucoma, or sleep apnea. Before taking any sleep remedy, talk to your physician first about possible side effects and harmful drug interactions.

DOING THINGS IN NEW WAYS

Having RA sometimes means that you must perform things a little differently than you did before you got sick. You might need to change the way you do your job. You may need more time in the morning to get dressed. Maybe you'll need to spend more time sitting when you prepare a meal.

At the heart of all of these changes is the important goal of preserving your joints. Inflamed joints are at greater risk for injury, so it's critical that you pay attention to how you use them. Though it might seem awkward at first to pause and think about how to open a can of soup, you will be rewarded down the road with less pain and stiffness. Even when your RA goes into remission, it's a good idea to remain vigilant about protecting your joints. Below are some tips that will make it easier for you to perform routine activities.

Self-Care
- Choose toothbrushes and hairbrushes with larger grips. Make them even larger by wrapping them in soft foam rubber or a foam hair curler.
- Choose clothes with Velcro closures rather than difficult buttons and snaps. Opt for clothing that is loose, with large necks and armholes.

- Avoid ironing by choosing clothes that don't need it.
- Wear slip-on shoes whenever possible.
- Use a long-handled shoehorn to help you slide into your shoes without having to bend down.
- Avoid hanging anything off your wrist, such as a purse.
- Sit down if you have to while drying your hair, applying makeup, or shaving.

Cooking

- When stirring foods, place your thumb on top of the spoon, as if you were stabbing at something. This position enables you to stir with your shoulder and reduces the pressure on your hands and wrists.
- Sit down to peel or cut vegetables and meats.
- Use an electric can opener instead of a manual one.
- Use a slotted spoon to remove food from boiling water rather than emptying a whole pot into the sink.
- Switch hands while cooking and stirring to alleviate stress on one hand.
- Purchase precut fruits and vegetables to reduce the time you spend cutting.
- Look for recipes that don't involve too many ingredients or the use of too many pots and pans.

Housecleaning

- If at all possible, hire someone else to do the cleaning and limit yourself to the maintenance duties.
- Sit down to fold and sort clean laundry.
- Wheel your cleaning supplies from room to room in a cart.
- Delegate cleanup tasks to other family members.
- When you do clean, take frequent breaks.
- Use spray cleaners to break down stains and debris, so you don't need to scrub as much.

- Make a realistic assessment of your cleaning needs. Do you really need to do as much as you're doing? Could the time be more wisely spent with friends and family or resting as needed?

Other Activities

- Avoid wringing and twisting motions. Let towels hang dry, or ask someone else to wring them out.
- Do not lean your body weight on your hands or wrists.
- Delegate tasks to other family members.
- Don't grip anything too tightly.
- When carrying heavy objects, keep them as close to your body as possible, so your spine can support your shoulders, elbows, and wrists.
- When getting up from a sitting position, slide forward as far as you can, then lean forward over your knees and swing up. Push off with your palms or forearms, making sure not to use your fingers.

ADDED ASSISTANCE

Sometimes, it isn't enough to do things a little differently. Sometimes, your joints may need some added support, which can come in the form of equipment specifically designed to protect your joints.

The Use of Splints

When a joint is inflamed, you may need to use a splint to stabilize it. A splint works by immobilizing the joint and ensuring it has maximal rest. Today's splints are typically made with a combination of plastic and fabric. They can be purchased in a drugstore, supermarket, or medical supplies store, or custom-fit by an occupational therapist. While a splint cannot prevent deformity, it can improve function and lessen pain and inflammation. Overusing a splint can cause stiffness and reduce strength and motion.

Assistive Equipment or Aids

Sometimes, when your pain is severe or movement is extremely difficult, you may need the help of assistive equipment such as a shower bench, a raised toilet seat, an elevated seat with armrests, or a walking cane. But use these assistive devices only if necessary. Overuse can eventually weaken the muscle and hurt the joint.

A Note on Footwear

When arthritis affects the feet, it can be difficult to find comfortable shoes. Swelling and stretched ligaments can cause the feet to widen and the toes to get higher. Wearing shoes that fit properly is one way to protect sensitive feet and prevent deformity.

Never buy a shoe in the hopes that it will stretch out and fit later on. Choose shoes that are lightweight and deep enough to accommodate the top of your toes. Make sure the shoes are wide enough, so that your toes don't pinch together. Also, put aside fashion and stick with sensible shoes with heels no higher than an inch. Wear shoes that offer good support on the inside of the foot as well as strong support in the back.

People who have deformities of the feet may require an insert to alleviate the pain in sensitive areas. If you're experiencing pressure on the ball of your foot, a metatarsal bar, which is an extra piece of rubber or leather, may be applied to the outside sole of the shoe. If you have severe deformities in your feet, you may need to order specially made shoes that are designed from a cast of your feet.

While you're coping with the pain and pressure of arthritic feet, make sure to practice good foot hygiene. Cut toenails straight across to avoid ingrown toenails. Keep your feet clean and dry, especially between the toes, and be on the lookout for blisters and sores. You can always see a podiatrist to help you cope with any symptoms that are particular to your feet.

WORKING WITH RA

It's sad but true: RA can take a toll on your ability to hold down a job and can affect your wage-earning potential. According to research by the Arthritis Research Center Foundation, people who have RA lose approximately $3,800 in annual wages compared to healthy peers of the same age, sex, and employment status. When adjusted for educational status, they had a wage loss of about $5,200.

But because RA is so variable, it's difficult to know the toll your condition will take on how you function on the job. If your case is mild, it may have no impact on your ability to work. If your job is physically demanding, you may experience some limitations. If you have a severe case of RA, you may have difficulty working at all.

The good news is that if you do become disabled by your condition, you are legally protected under the Americans with Disabilities Act (ADA), a law passed by Congress in 1990. The ADA prohibits employers with fifteen or more employees from discriminating against people with disabilities in making decisions about hiring and employment. In addition to employment, the law guarantees equal opportunity in transportation, public accommodations, state and local government services, and telecommunications. Other employment protections afforded by the ADA include the following:

- In the event you do need certain accommodations, your employer cannot pay you a lower wage or salary to cover the cost of these accommodations. An employer also can't ask you to pay for these items. If any modification poses undue economic hardship on the employer, the company must offer you the option of providing it yourself or paying for part of it.
- An employer cannot ask if you have a disability or about the severity of it. But an employer is allowed to ask if you are able to perform the essential duties of the job.

- Before offering you a job, an employer cannot ask you to have a medical examination. After a job offer, however, the employer can make that request provided all employees in that position are required to do the same. Your medical records must remain confidential.
- Your employer must offer you the same health insurance benefits that are offered to other employees. But an employer is not required to offer you extra benefits to cover your medical condition.
- If it's obvious that you have a disability that will interfere with—or already does affect—your ability to perform certain tasks, your employer is entitled to ask you to describe or demonstrate how you would perform the tasks and whether you need any accommodations to help you do them.

The ADA does not require employers to:

- Make major changes to accommodate your condition. The law specifically notes that employers do not need to provide accommodations that impose "undue hardship" on business operations.
- Lower their quality and production standards to accommodate your disability.
- Provide personal-use items such as splints or special eyewear for people with disabilities.

To Tell or Not to Tell

According to the Arthritis Foundation, your decision on whether or not to tell your employer you have RA could be based on three factors: whether it's obvious you have a disability, whether you need special accommodations in order to do your job, and the effort it will take for you to keep your RA a secret.

It's important to think it through before deciding to discuss your condition with your employer. If you work for a corporation with a strong commitment to helping the disabled and making necessary accommodations, you could benefit from telling your employer. Perhaps you can work out a new schedule, or maybe you can shift from a full-time job to a part-time one. Maybe your employer would gladly support your wish to do a job share with another employee.

But if you do bring up your condition, you're likely to raise questions about your ability to do your job. You may also worry that you won't be considered for future promotions, plum positions, and special assignments. In addition, you may be concerned that prospective employers will dismiss you as a job candidate for fear of high medical bills. You may wonder, too, whether your coworkers will treat you differently. All of these concerns are bona fide worries and factors you should consider before deciding to reveal your medical condition to your employer and colleagues.

The inability to perform a job you were once proficient at can be stressful, frustrating, and harmful to your health. So if you are having trouble doing your job, consider speaking with a vocational rehabilitation counselor or social worker. These professionals can help assess your marketable skills and assist in your decision about whether to stay with your current job, find a new job, or train for a new and different profession.

If you do decide to tell your employer you have RA, choose a time when neither of you is under undue pressure or stress. Describe your condition in simple terms and explain how it might affect your work. Explain that you are not looking for sympathy, but rather for ways to resolve these difficulties that will benefit both you and your employer. It's a good idea to research the kinds of changes you are looking for beforehand. Keep in mind that this may be your employer's first encounter with RA, so you may be educating him about the disease. Being open and honest about your life and needs—within reason to your privacy—will allow you to come up with solutions rather than isolate you with more problems.

On the Job

Assume you have just learned you have RA and are starting to experience some pain and fatigue. Whether or not you decide to share that information with your employer, you might find that you need to start doing your job a little differently. Here are some tips:

- Pace your workload. Alternate between light tasks and heavy ones.
- Create an efficient work space. Place things you use frequently within easy reach, so that you minimize lifting, carrying, and reaching.
- Sit down to do most tasks, if you can.
- If you work at a desk job, make sure your computer, chair, and desk are at appropriate heights. Consult with an occupational therapist or ergonomics expert, if necessary.
- Take regular breaks—especially when you feel your joints stiffening—and do some gentle stretches.
- Trade off tasks that stress your joints with a coworker.
- Use modified tools and equipment, if necessary, such as pens with thick handles.
- Talk to your employer about the possibility of working hours when you feel most energetic.
- Finally, be honest with yourself about your ability to do your job. Remember, your health must be a priority.

What If You Become Disabled?

There's no doubt that having RA can cause disability. A Finnish survey of patients with established RA found that RA patients were nearly eight times more likely to report moderate disability than people who did not have RA.

If you do become disabled, you may be eligible for Social Security disability benefits. The Social Security Administration considers a person disabled if he or she is unable to do any kind of work for which he or she is suited, if the disability is expected to last at least a year, or if it could result in death. The two types of benefits are Social Security Disability Insurance and Supplemental Security Income.

Fortunately, not everyone who has RA is destined to become disabled. A Swedish study that followed 168 RA patients for ten years or more found that 94 percent of them continued to be independent in their daily activities, and only 10 percent reported having serious disability. Clearly, people who have RA are no longer doomed to a wheelchair. And with the new medications available to treat RA, fewer and fewer people are even winding up disabled.

TRAVELING WITH RA

When your body is wracked with the pain of RA and you're feeling overwhelmed by the fatigue, the thought of taking a trip might be the furthest thing from your mind. But imagine lounging poolside at a Caribbean resort, shopping and sightseeing in a historic town, or taking in a beautiful sunset at your favorite beach. Escaping to a beloved getaway could be just what the doctor ordered.

Having RA doesn't mean the end of traveling. It simply means you'll need to adapt your plans to accommodate your condition. It means smart planning, so you'll remember your medications and any other special devices you use. It means strategizing, so that you don't overdo it and tire yourself out. It might mean adjusting your vacation plans a bit so that you don't choose a destination that saps your energy. For instance, while hiking steep mountains may have been your vacation of choice in the past, you might have to choose less rigorous outings now.

Here are some tips to keep your vacation plans as stress-free as possible:

- If you're planning to fly, make reservations early. Consider requesting your seat assignment when you book the flight. Ask for seating that provides more legroom, such as a seat in the first row or one in an exit row.
- When flying, always keep medications and other personal items with you in the event there is a delay or your luggage is lost.
- If you have an artificial joint, an implant, or a metal shoe insert, consider bringing a letter from your doctor. These devices may trigger the new, more sensitive metal detection equipment at the airport, and a letter from your doctor could explain the situation.
- If you're using a self-injectable RA medication, be sure to bring a letter from your physician. Some airports now have new security regulations that may require people traveling with syringes and needles to provide proof that the supplies are medically necessary.
- Travel as light as possible. Avoid overpacking your luggage. Bring less clothing and plan to do laundry on your trip. Call hotels ahead of time to find out if they have certain amenities that you can leave at home, such as blow-dryers.
- Invest in lightweight luggage on wheels.
- Try to book a nonstop direct flight to avoid the inconvenience of transferring to another plane in an unfamiliar airport. If you have no choice, find out how long it will take you to get to your connecting flight. Then request additional time between your flights when booking your ticket,

or make arrangements to get there by way of an electric cart. Additionally, if you are on a flight for a long time, be sure to move around and stand as much as possible. Sitting still for too long can cause circulation issues.

- Always wear comfortable shoes. Long lines are common at airports and train stations, so you'll want to be dressed in your most comfortable footwear.
- Don't hesitate to ask for help. If you have difficulty walking long distances, ask for assistance at the airport. Some airports provide electric carts or trams to take you to the gate. If you notify the airline forty-eight hours ahead of your flight, you can also arrange to have a wheelchair.
- If possible, avoid traveling at peak times of the day like the morning and late afternoon, when airports and train stations are at their busiest.
- Do your research. If traveling by train, find out whether bathrooms are handicapped accessible. And if you use a wheelchair, find out if you can get assistance from train personnel with boarding and exiting, and whether you can board in advance.
- Preboard on flights. Most airlines will allow passengers with disabilities or in wheelchairs to board in advance.
- Take travel breaks to prevent stiffness. On a flight or on a train, do some simple range-of-motion exercises, and get up for some walking and stretching. If you're traveling by car, make frequent stops, so you can get out and stretch.
- Bring a light snack. If you need to take your medications with food, it's always wise to have something to eat with you. That way you don't need to wait for snacks to be served or venture through a moving train to the food service car.
- Whether traveling by airplane, train, or car, consider bringing a horseshoe pillow for head and neck support.

- Adapt your vehicle. Install special wide-angle side-view and rearview mirrors to increase your field of view without having to twist and turn around in the driver's seat. Use a cushioned seat belt for greater shoulder comfort. Cover your steering wheel in sheepskin so you can use a looser grip and protect your hand joints.
- If you're traveling by car, consider using pillows and cushions for support and pain relief. Cervical collars can help lessen neck pain, while a lumbar pillow can provide lower-back support. You can also use cushions for a sore back or hips.
- Once you're at your destination, take time to rest and relax. Make leisure and relaxation a priority, and continue to take care of your health.

A FINAL NOTE

Living with a chronic disease like RA is not easy. But it doesn't have to deter you from living an enjoyable and productive life. The key is to modify your lifestyle, so that you minimize your pain and fatigue and preserve the integrity of your joints. Don't be afraid to ask others for help. Whether it's calling a social worker for advice on finding new employment or asking your spouse to take on more of the housework, speaking up for yourself is critical to self-care.

PROFILE

DIANE

As a young child, Diane witnessed her mother's suffering from rheumatoid arthritis. "I saw the damage it did to her over the years," Diane recalls. "They didn't have the meds that are available today; she grinned and bared it all. She fought the long fight showing a kind of strength I could only hope to emulate."

At fourteen, Diane began her own lifelong battle with RA. She had pain from head to toe, she recalls, and the joints in her knees, elbows, ankles, and hands were hot and swollen. She felt stiff and lost the exuberant energy of a normal, healthy teenager. "I woke up one morning feeling as if I had a lead weighted body cast on," she says. "I could barely get out of bed. My entire body slowed down. My joints began to stiffen but with very little pain. The pain came days later."

A year later, Diane went into remission without the help of medication. She even joined the high school drill team. In her twenties, she got pregnant with her daughter and remained pain-free. But in her thirties, the pain returned. She was raising her daughter, finishing school, and working a job. But Diane vowed she would not give in to the disease. "I promised myself that I would not end up in a wheelchair or in a corner wasting away if I could help it," she says.

She began experimenting with different drugs like Relafen, an NSAID, and Azulfidine, a disease-modifying antirheumatic drug (DMARD). When her liver enzymes were thrown off, she had to find a new regimen.

Now forty-six, she takes a combination of Arava, Plaquenil, and methotrexate. "It's a combination that seems to be working," she says. "I can stand up straight when I get out of bed."

RA has definitely taken a toll on her job. As coordinator of a parenting skills program for a social services agency, she can no longer drive because her ankles are unreliable. If she wants to make a community presentation, she has to make special transportation arrangements and limit the amount of program materials she carries. She limits her work on the computer to no more than twenty minutes at a stretch, and gives her hands and wrists frequent rests.

"I also have to plan my work/life schedule around maintaining a balance of work and rest, or at the very least the fatigue will hit me like an invisible brick," she says. "Then, even my brain slows down."

What troubles her most is that she always has to consider whether she can physically handle an assignment. "I feel awful sometimes because I don't want to seem like a slacker," she says. "But I don't want to be unsuccessful either because a body part failed me."

Even more challenging is the fact that she looks healthy. "To everyone who looks at me, the response is, 'Well, you look okay,'" Diane says. "Well, I do look okay until you take a closer look at my hands with the extra-large knuckles, the arms that have a permanent bend in them, and the wrists that have limited flexibility."

To help her endure the pain of RA, she has modified her home to make it more RA friendly. She eliminated excess clutter, so she has less to clean and arrange. She stores food items in small quantities, so the containers stay light. She cooks several meals at a time, so she spends less time on her feet. To spare her of excess trips, Diane stores cleaning products upstairs and downstairs. She uses easy-grip utensils and long-handled cleaning brushes, too.

In addition to working with a good doctor, Diane goes to great lengths to stay healthy. She regularly scans the Internet for useful information about her condition and ways to strengthen her body, spirit, and mind. As an avid fan of healthy eating, she has reduced her intake of salt, sugar, and simple carbohydrates, and increased her intake of water. She also takes fish oil supplements and a multivitamin every day.

Exercising every day at home, she says, helps her stay physically strong. Her routines vary and may include yoga, aerobics, Pilates, and light weight lifting. After her workouts, Diane likes to meditate, which helps her keep stress in check. When she meditates, she takes time to acknowledge how her body feels, so she knows what it needs.

She also finds it helpful to have conversations with other people who have RA, to hear their experiences, and to trade practical tips on coping. Her boss has RA, too, and so completely understands Diane's challenges. "Talking with people who are moving forward in their lives despite RA makes me feel less alone," she says. She enjoys reading about others with RA in magazines like *Arthritis Today*.

Over the years, Diane has become better about asking for help. At home, she asks her husband and daughter to help her in and out of the bathtub when she's in the mood for a bath. At work, she asks colleagues for help in lifting things or twisting off the cap on a bottle of juice. At the supermarket, she asks the clerks to pack the bags lightly. Her husband now does all of the laundry and helps with grocery shopping. "It was hard at first to ask for help at the store, in the office, or even at home," she says. "But as I've become more comfortable with myself, that has become easier."

These experiences, coupled with a strong inner spirit and memories of her mother's strength, she says, are what keep her moving forward, even on her worst days. "When I experience a flare-up, sometimes for a moment, just a moment, I want to die," she says. "Then I hear a whisper from my spirit, which tells me, 'Not yet.'"

Instead, Diane tries to focus her energies on what she enjoys about life by writing in her journal. "I have cried for the loss of what I can no longer do, but I have to know that that was my life then, and this is now. Then I take a deep appreciating breath and smile. I'm here alive."

CHAPTER FIVE ❧

Eating Well with RA

In an ideal world, we'd be able to suggest an eating strategy that alleviates all the pain, inflammation, and fatigue associated with RA. We'd have a tailored exercise plan that would make you feel less stiff, eliminate the achiness in your joints, and restore you to your pre-RA mobility. Unfortunately, no such diet or exercise plans exist. There are no magical foods that can cause the inflammation to subside, no special vitamins or minerals that can reduce the pain, and no exceptional exercise routines that will permanently take away the symptoms of RA.

Does that mean you should ignore your diet? Or abandon your efforts to exercise? Not at all. A key part of managing your RA is attaining a healthy weight, and eating a healthy diet and getting exercise are critical components in that effort. Excess weight puts extra pressure on your joints, which only worsens your pain and causes more fatigue. Giving up exercise will further reduce your muscle mass, causing even more weakness in your joints. That's why having RA makes it even more important to eat well and exercise. We'll start this chapter with a discussion of nutrition.

NUTRITION BASICS

The notion that a special diet can affect RA and its symptoms is an appealing one indeed. For decades, researchers have been trying to find a connection between diet and arthritis. So far, there is nothing that confirms that any particular diet, or even food, can help or hurt RA. But that hasn't stopped unscrupulous manufacturers from peddling remedies—dietary and otherwise—that promise a quick fix for arthritis.

Healthy eating should be part of everyone's routine, whether or not they have a chronic disease. Unfortunately, most Americans have gotten away from good nutrition and eat diets laden with excess calories, fat, sugar, and salt. They order extra-large portions in fast-food restaurants, eat meals on the run, and indulge in high-calorie treats at the expense of healthier options such as fruits and vegetables.

Now that you have RA, it's important to get a handle on your eating habits. Let's start with a brief primer on the major components in your diet and other important nutrients.

Carbohydrates

In recent years, carbohydrates have been demonized by the food industry as the villain behind America's weight gain, spawning an entire industry of low-carb foods. Diets like the one created by the late Dr. Robert Atkins told Americans to ditch the carbs and keep the fats, allowing room for foods like bacon, sausage, and cheese.

But in reality, carbohydrates are a critical component of a healthy diet and the body's preferred and primary source of energy. In fact, the American Dietetic Association (ADA) recommends that carbohydrates make up at least 50 percent of your daily diet. The ADA also advises that consumers beware of eating low-carb foods in an effort to lose weight; just because a food is low in carbohydrates doesn't mean it's low in calories.

The problem isn't that Americans are eating too many carbo-hydrates, but rather that they're eating the wrong kind. Carbohydrates come in two forms: simple and complex. Simple carbohydrates are found naturally in fruits, vegetables, and milk, but are also found in foods that contain refined sugars, which have been processed to extract natural sucrose found in plants to sweeten the flavor. Nutritionally, refined sugars are considered empty calories, foods that provide energy but no nutrients, vita-mins, or minerals. Once digested, these simple carbohydrates break down rapidly into simple sugars.

Complex carbohydrates are starches and fiber found in legumes, grains, and vegetables. Starch is derived from the storage systems of plants, such as beans, lentils, potatoes, wheat, and oats. Like the sugars found in simple carbohydrates, starches break down into simple sugars, but they do so much more slowly.

Fiber, on the other hand, cannot be digested in the stomach at all because humans lack the enzymes to break it down. Fiber comes in two varieties: soluble and insoluble. Soluble fibers can dissolve in water and are found in dried peas and beans, apples, carrots, and oats. Although the exact mechanism is unclear, soluble fibers slow the time it takes to empty the stomach. They also lower cholesterol levels. The fiber binds to bile acids, which are made of cholesterol, and transports them out of the body as waste.

Insoluble fibers, also called roughage, do not dissolve in water and are found in whole wheat foods, green beans, wheat bran, and broccoli. Because insoluble fibers absorb water, they can add bulk to the stool and help move food through the digestive tract.

Proteins

Unlike carbohydrates and fats, proteins are generally held in high regard for their role in building muscle and strength. But in fact, protein has numerous roles in our bodies. Besides providing structure to our bodies, protein is necessary to build and repair body tissues. Proteins also have a major role in regulating body processes, and exist in our bodies in various forms as enzymes, hormones, and antibodies. They also assist in the transport of important molecules and the contraction of muscles, and aid in fluid balance, acid balance, and nerve transmission. In the absence of enough carbohydrates or fat, protein serves as a source of energy.

Proteins come from various sources, including eggs, meat, and milk. Plant sources of protein include legumes such as lentils, chickpeas, and black beans, as well as nuts and seeds.

Fats

The melt-in-your-mouth sensation of a bite of cheesecake owes its smooth, mouthwatering effects to fat. Fat is also what makes a chocolate bar so creamy, fried chicken so crispy, and Grandma's cookies so light and airy.

Like carbohydrates, fats have been held in low esteem as the culprit behind America's rapidly expanding waistline. But in reality, fats are an essential part of our diet, too. They play important roles in the functioning of the brain and nervous system. They allow our bodies to use fat-soluble vitamins A, D, E, and K, and help insulate our bodies from cold temperatures. Fat also acts as a protective cushion for your internal organs. As a source of energy, fat delivers nine calories per gram, compared with four calories per gram for carbohydrates and proteins.

Fat comes in two basic forms: saturated and unsaturated. Saturated fats, which are unhealthy in large amounts, are solid at room temperature and come from meat, whole-milk dairy products, butter, and palm and coconut oils. A diet rich in saturated fats can clog arteries and raise your risk for heart disease.

Unsaturated fats are the healthier fats and come in two forms. The monounsaturated variety comes from nuts, avocados, and olive oil. Polyunsaturated fats are liquids found mostly in vegetable oils, such as safflower, sunflower, and corn. They are also found in fish in the form of omega-3 fatty acids.

Research has suggested that the omega-3 fatty acids found in fish oils can reduce the pain and swelling of RA. In studies, two specific acids—eicosapentaenoic acid (EPA) and docosahexaenoic acid (DHA)—have been shown to reduce morning stiffness and the number of swollen joints. However, there is no research showing that fish oil supplements are superior to nonsteroidal anti-inflammatory drugs for relieving pain or that fish oil can slow the progression of disease.

If you do decide to take fish oil supplements, talk to your doctor first. Fish oil has a blood-thinning effect. Combining it with NSAIDs, aspirin, or blood-thinning medications such as warfarin or heparin may cause excessive bleeding. In addition, some fish oils may be high in fat-soluble vitamins, which can cause toxic effects in the body if allowed to build up. A better way to increase your intake of omega-3 fatty acids is simply to eat more cold-water fish, which include salmon, sardines, mackerel, herring, anchovy, and lake trout.

Some unsaturated fats are processed to make them stable and solid at room temperature with the addition of hydrogen, a process called hydrogenation. This process can produce trans fatty acids, which have been linked to high cholesterol and heart disease. Foods that contain trans fatty acids are difficult to avoid. Hydrogenated and partially hydrogenated oils are used in all kinds of processed foods, including breakfast cereals, frozen waffles, granola bars, potato chips, cookies, crackers, and more. They are also found in margarine and shortening.

IMPORTANT VITAMINS AND MINERALS

Many vitamins and minerals play critical roles in keeping us healthy. Certain ones deserve some special attention for the role they have in RA.

Calcium

RA increases your risk for having osteoporosis, a disease in which the bones become increasingly thin and brittle. If you have had RA for a long time, take corticosteroid medications such as prednisone, and are slight of build, your risk for osteoporosis goes up. You're also at risk if you are female, have a family history of osteoporosis, and are unable to get adequate amounts of physical activity.

Calcium, a mineral found in milk, yogurt, cheese, broccoli, and spinach, helps counter the breakdown of bone. In children and young adults, calcium builds and strengthens bones. In adults, calcium continues to strengthen bones and slows the rate of bone loss that occurs with age. Calcium also plays a role in the contraction of muscles, including that of the heart, and in nerve function and blood clotting.

Phosphorus

The second most important mineral for bones is phosphorus. Together with calcium, phosphorus makes up the solid mineral deposit of bone and teeth. This omnipresent mineral can be found in virtually all foods, but is most prevalent in protein-rich foods such as milk, meat, poultry, fish, eggs, legumes, and nuts.

Vitamin D

Known as the sunshine vitamin, vitamin D is essential for the absorption of calcium and phosphorus. Milk fortified with vitamin D is a good source. It can also be manufactured in the skin when you're exposed to sunlight. Preliminary research suggests that vitamin D may have a protective role in RA. It may also play a role in alleviating joint and muscle pain in patients who are vitamin D deficient.

Folic Acid

In recent years, folic acid has gotten attention for its role in preventing neural tube defects in unborn babies. But folic acid also plays an important role in manufacturing new body cells, and it works with vitamin B12 to produce hemoglobin in red blood cells. In addition, folic acid lowers levels of homocysteine, an amino acid that has been associated with heart disease.

Folic acid, also called folate or folacin, can be found in leafy vegetables, legumes, certain fruits, and fortified cereals. Enriched grain products, such as macaroni, bread, cornmeal, rice, and flour are also fortified with folic acid. People who take methotrexate to treat RA may be at risk for deficiency of folic acid and require supplementation.

The Antioxidant Vitamins

Antioxidants—vitamin C, vitamin E, and beta-carotene, which forms vitamin A—are believed to shield the body from free-oxygen radicals that cause disease. Experts believe that people who have RA have excessive amounts of free-oxygen radicals in their joints, which causes the joint damage. Antioxidants, some research suggests, may counter this destruction by neutralizing these free-oxygen radicals and converting them into harmless waste products.

One recent study found that vitamin C can actually help prevent RA. The study found that people who ate the least amount of fruits and vegetables were twice as likely to develop inflammation in the joints compared with people who ate the most.

Beta-carotene and vitamin C are found in fruits and vegetables. Vitamin E is found in vegetable oils, nuts, and grains.

Vitamin B6

People who have RA tend to have lower levels of vitamin B6, or pyridoxine, a B vitamin found in whole grain cereals, fish, bananas, and peanut butter. One study found that as levels of vitamin B6 decreased, the activity, severity, and pain of RA increased.

Having low levels of vitamin B6 makes it hard for your body to adequately break down an amino acid called homocysteine, which has been associated with heart disease and stroke. Experts believe it's the inflammation in RA that causes a reduction in vitamin B6, suggesting that people with RA may need more of the vitamin to prevent a deficiency.

WEIGHT AND RA

Having RA can make it hard to achieve and maintain a healthy weight. The aches and pain may become so overwhelming that you can no longer prepare a healthy meal and now rely increasingly on prepackaged meals. Or maybe you no longer have the strength to do any physical activity to burn off excess calories. Certain medications like steroids can also make you prone to weight gain.

But maintaining a healthy weight is important for people who have RA. Excess weight taxes the body's weight-bearing joints, which can cause more pain. Being too thin can make you weak and put your bones at risk. The goal, then, is to eat a healthy diet and to try to keep your weight within a healthy range.

Healthy Eating

With two-thirds of the population overweight, many Americans are fighting a constant battle against weight gain. Achieving a healthy weight and staying there may take practice and require modifying old habits.

While there is no specific diet for an RA patient to follow, there are important guidelines that can help anyone eat more healthfully. Experts offer the following tips:

- Eat a variety of foods. Choose foods from the different food groups—bread, cereal, rice, and pasta; vegetables and fruit; dairy products; and lean or low-fat meat. Remember, no one food can make you fat if it's eaten in moderation.

- Avoid foods rich in saturated fat and cholesterol. Switch from high-fat foods to the low-fat version. Select meats that are lower in fat, or try eating seafood a couple of times a week. Opt for low-fat or skim milk instead of whole milk. Making these simple switches cuts calories and fat.
- Drink plenty of fluids, especially water. Staying well-hydrated helps sustain normal body functions. Also, limit your intake of soda, which is full of sugar and contains no healthful nutrients.
- Restrict your intake of refined sugar and sodium. Sugary substances generally come with plenty of calories but have little nutritional value. Eating too much salt can also raise blood pressure.
- Drink alcohol only in moderation. Alcohol supplies seven calories per gram and also can stimulate the appetite. Patients who are taking methotrexate should not drink alcohol at all.
- Fill up on grains, vegetables, and fruits. These foods are generally higher in fiber and lower in calories. They also contain more vitamins and minerals and can help curb your appetite. Aim to eat at least five servings of fruits or vegetables a day.

If you're actively trying to lose weight, try adopting some of the following habits from the ADA:

- Plan meals and snacks ahead of time. Pack a healthy lunch for work, and keep healthy snacks on hand wherever you are.
- Purchase food on a full stomach. You'll be less tempted to buy high-fat, high-calorie foods if you're not hungry.
- Eat slowly. Savor each bite, and allow time for the food to reach your stomach. It takes about twenty minutes for your stomach to tell your brain that it's full.

- Check portion sizes. Use smaller bowls and dinner plates so your servings look larger. Place the food directly on your plate rather than serving it in bowls and platters on the table.
- Make eating the focus of a meal. Sit down and focus on your food, rather than nibbling mindlessly while doing other tasks. Eating while watching TV or driving can lead you to eat more.
- Stop eating when the meal is over. Don't eat leftovers off your child's plate or nibble while you're cleaning up.
- Be on the lookout for emotional eating. Avoid eating when you're bored, depressed, or stressed. Find other, more active ways to release these emotions.

Risk for Malnutrition

Weight gain is just one problem that people with RA may experience. Patients with RA may also be at greater risk for being underweight. One study found that as many as 26 percent of RA patients are malnourished. The chronic inflammation associated with RA spurs the production of cytokines, such as interleukin-1 and tumor necrosis factor, which increases the body's metabolic rate and protein breakdown. At the same time, the patient is experiencing pain, which can make it a challenge to prepare and eat food, especially if the patient lives alone.

Weight loss may also result because extra energy is needed to fight off fever. But the accompanying aches and pain of RA may suppress the appetite, making it difficult to satisfy the additional energy needs.

If you're having a hard time maintaining your weight, follow these tips from the ADA:

- Eat more frequent meals. Try eating five or six small meals a day instead of two or three large ones.

- Focus on nutrient-rich foods and beverages. Ditch the diet sodas for milk and milk shakes.
- Look for ways to stimulate your appetite. Fill the house with mouthwatering aromas. Keep favorite foods handy. Add texture, aroma, and color to your foods.
- Eat when it's time. Rather than wait for hunger cues, follow the clock for guidance. When it's time to eat, indulge.
- Steer clear of unpleasant subjects and thoughts before eating, especially if you're prone to stress.

OTHER DIETS

In an era when nutrition is regularly in the news, it's tempting to look for ways to manipulate our diets to relieve aches and pain. People who have RA may be especially eager to try new ways of eating in the quest for pain relief. Here are two strategies you may hear about.

Elimination Diets

Although there's no scientific evidence to back it up, many people believe that certain foods and food additives can worsen their arthritis pain. Foods that potentially aggravate RA pain include tomatoes, corn, pork, oranges, milk, and foods that contain gluten.

If you suspect that a certain food is making your RA symptoms worse, you may consider trying an elimination diet. Removing a food from your diet, then gradually reintroducing it in small quantities may help you identify a food culprit. But if you do want to try an elimination diet, talk to your doctor or a registered dietitian first. Eliminating a food that supplies important nutrients—the calcium and vitamin D in milk, for instance—means that you'll need to use supplements or another food to replace the nutrients you're taking out.

Fasting

Some research has suggested that fasting can relieve the symptoms of RA. One study from Norway found that patients with RA who underwent seven to ten days of fasting, then followed it up with a gluten-free vegan diet for three and a half months experienced a positive effect. But experts agree that the benefits of fasting are short-lived, and that fasting is a high-risk way to treat RA pain.

FINALLY: PATIENTS BEWARE

The pain and frustration associated with RA makes patients who have this disease easy targets for unscrupulous marketers promising a quick dietary fix. The bottom line is this: At this time, there is no scientific evidence to back up any diet in the treatment of RA. Your best bet is to eat a well-balanced diet, filled with good foods that help you achieve a healthy weight.

PROFILE

ROSEMARY

The first symptoms of rheumatoid arthritis emerged shortly after Rosemary had given birth to her second child. Pains in her wrists and hands surfaced during an exercise class, and Rosemary knew that something was wrong.

Almost immediately, at the age of twenty-nine, Rosemary was diagnosed with RA. "Even when the doctor had the 'I'm so sorry' look on his face, I was in denial, or maybe ignorant, of the impact the disease would have on my future," she says.

She was sent to a rheumatologist, who promptly put her on aspirin therapy. Every day, she took twelve coated aspirins. "Fortunately, I'm blessed with a cast-iron stomach," she says.

A holistic healer suggested that her disease was the result of a systemic yeast infection, so Rosemary decided to eliminate all sugars and foods that contained yeast from her diet. Rosemary did go into remission shortly after that, but she credits it to the fact that she got pregnant, not to the fact that she ate a sugar- and yeast-free diet. Once she was more or less pain-free, she stopped seeing the healer and ditched the diet.

But after the birth of her fourth child, the symptoms returned. Her joints ached, and she awoke feeling stiff almost every morning. "I guess the only option for me was to stay pregnant," she quips.

Rosemary experimented with sulfasalazine and Plaquenil, until she started taking her current regimen of methotrexate, Enbrel, and Relafen. The combination definitely helps reduce her pain, though she continues to live every single day with some sort of pain and discomfort. She tries to alleviate the pain with the use of heating pads or warm cups of tea, which usually do the trick.

But it's the fatigue, she says, that bothers her most of all. "I would love to be a person with high energy, but I'm just not," she says. "It's not fun to live with the fatigue. I used to think, 'Oh, it's because I'm middle-aged.' And some nights, I definitely lose sleep if the pain is bad and wakes me up. But it's not just age or loss of sleep. It's the arthritis itself. People don't think that having arthritis causes fatigue, but fatigue is a true side effect of having rheumatoid arthritis."

Though after twenty-one years she's become accustomed to having RA, the fifty-year-old stay-at-home mother of four says the disease colors every single aspect of her life. Turning the ignition to start the car used to be painful. Opening jars remains a challenge. And as a one-time high school athlete—she still manages to walk about fifteen miles a week—she desperately wishes that she could be more physical. "I really wish I could show my son my sweet jump shot, but a basketball is too heavy for my wrist," she says.

Having RA also affects the way she interprets everything that happens to her health. Just recently, Rosemary was having problems with her kidneys. Right away, she was convinced that it was kidney damage, caused by years of using such powerful medications. Her doctor was suspicious too, and immediately took Rosemary off all three of her RA medications.

Two weeks later, after the medication in her system had dissipated, Rosemary was wracked with pain again. As it turns out, all she really had was a run-of-the-mill kidney infection, which had nothing to do with the RA.

Rosemary used the opportunity to try to cut back on her medications. "I wanted to try going back on only the Enbrel injection and the nonsteroidal anti-inflammatory medication without the methotrexate," she says. "But there wasn't much power there. I need the methotrexate, and now I'm waiting for it to kick in." The experience, she says, taught her that she's willing to assume the risks from the medication in order to live with less pain.

Rosemary has also had surgeries as a result of her RA, one to correct symptoms of carpal tunnel syndrome, and another to fuse her thumb joint where the cartilage had completely eroded and the joint had become bone on bone. She fully anticipates that she will have more surgeries in the future, most probably on her feet and hands, where most of her pain is concentrated.

The key to managing her condition, Rosemary says, has been finding the right balance—the proper balance of rest and exercise and the best mix of medications. "I also know that with bad days there will also come good days," she says. "Sure there are some things that can't be done because of the physical limitations. But you just shift your focus to those things that can be done."

CHAPTER SIX ❧

Exercising with RA

Not many years ago, people who had RA were confined to bed rest. Sometimes, patients were even hospitalized in an effort to bring the disease under control. And in fact, rest did—and still does—help reduce inflammation and pain, which only confirmed the value of confining a patient to bed.

But what medical experts at the time failed to realize was that the lack of physical activity also caused muscles to weaken. Bones became increasingly fragile and brittle. The patient's overall fitness deteriorated.

Gradually, medical experts began to experiment with exercise in patients whose RA was under control. Their research found that not only could these patients do strengthening and low-impact aerobic exercises, but they actually derived a lot of benefits from movement. They became less fatigued, were better able to function, and had more energy.

Today, experts know that patients with RA need a healthy balance of both rest and exercise. Regular exercise improves strength and energy, increases the stability of your joints, prevents joint deformity, builds bone, and decreases pain. It also enhances your sleep, decreases stress and anxiety, and promotes self-esteem. Regular activity improves overall fitness, too, by strengthening the cardiovascular system, and helps promote weight loss and maintenance. At the same time, rest is important during a flare-up and to help your joints stabilize.

The key is to determine the right kinds and amount of exercise for you. Every patient is different. Some may be able to do more. Others may require more rest. By consulting with your physician and a physical therapist trained to work with arthritis patients, you can devise a custom exercise plan that will help improve your functioning.

GETTING OVER THE PAIN

When you're besieged by the pain of RA, exercise is probably the last thing on your mind. You might find it too difficult even to perform simple tasks like getting out of bed, climbing the stairs, and cooking a meal. But avoiding physical activity can put you on a vicious cycle. The less you move, the weaker and smaller your muscles become. And as your muscles get smaller and weaker, your joints will become stiffer and increasingly inflexible, making it even harder for you to get the physical activity you need.

The lack of exercise can also exacerbate depression, which is common among patients suffering from chronic pain. Feeling depressed, in turn, can make it harder to exercise. Again, you wind up trapped in a vicious cycle of pain, depression, and a lack of exercise.

That's why it's critical to do some physical activity, no matter how small or insignificant it may seem. Gardening, sweeping, and short walks around the block can make an enormous difference to a body that's been wracked with pain. Remember, it's best to talk to your rheumatologist or a physical therapist before beginning any exercise program. A trained physical therapist can provide specific exercises that suit your condition.

TYPES OF EXERCISE

Basically, there are three types of exercise, all of which can play a role in improving your symptoms. These are:

Strength Training

Not only for the muscle-bound, strength training benefits anyone who wants to maintain her vitality. For the patient with RA, strength training is an essential component of any exercise routine. Strength training builds muscles, which in turn helps support and protect the joints. Studies show that patients with RA who maintain a home-based strength-training routine are able to sustain that strength.

Certain types of strength training may be better than others for different patients. The types of strength training you should know include:

- **Isometrics.** These exercises require tightening or contracting a specific muscle without moving your joints. Your body, then, provides resistance to the muscle, and no special equipment is required. Isometrics are especially helpful when you first develop RA and when you're experiencing a painful flare-up. Some Pilates and yoga moves are isometric and can improve both strength and flexibility.
- **Isotonics.** These exercises combine joint movements with muscle resistance for a slightly more rigorous workout. Muscle resistance may involve the use of weights, exercise machines, elastic bands, or your own body weight. Because isotonics are more rigorous, they are generally reserved for patients who are not experiencing pain and inflammation; however, they build muscle faster than isometric exercise and thus you may see greater benefits over time. Lunges, squats, and biceps curls are all examples of isotonic moves.

- **Water resistance training.** A good way for RA patients to build strength is to perform exercises in a pool. The water provides resistance to the muscles at the same time that it gives support to the joints, making a water workout less likely to lead to injury and pain.

The National Institute of Arthritis and Musculoskeletal and Skin Diseases (NIAMS) recommends that you do strengthening exercises every other day unless you're experiencing severe swelling or pain in your joints.

Range-of-Motion Exercises

The ability to move freely without stiffness is the reward of range-of-motion exercises. This type of physical activity improves flexibility, helps sustain joint mobility, and reduces stiffness. Range-of-motion exercises involve moving each joint as far as it can go in each possible direction. Good examples of these types of exercises are stretches, yoga, and some Pilates moves. Joints that require range-of-motion exercises in RA patients include the fingers, hands, wrists, elbows, shoulders, hips, knees, ankles, and toes.

According to NIAMS, these exercises should be done once or twice a day, and whenever you feel your joints becoming stiff. To figure out exactly which exercises to do, talk to a physical therapist. One recent study found that tai chi, a martial art, may have range-of-motion benefits for RA patients. Although it doesn't appear to reduce pain or lessen the severity of disease, the patients experienced an improvement in the range of motion in the joints of their legs and ankles, and also reported greater enjoyment of exercise.

Cardiovascular Exercises

Activities that improve the strength of your heart and its ability to beat stronger for longer periods of time are considered cardiovascular exercises. When you engage in cardiovascular exercises, you breathe harder, so your heart and lungs are working harder, too. These exercises also improve blood flow, burn calories, and lower blood pressure, triglycerides, and LDL cholesterol, the bad cholesterol. At the same time, they help raise HDL cholesterol, which is the good kind. Before doing any cardiovascular exercise, check with your physician. Your doctor can tell you if you are adopting a safe and acceptable regimen for you. For example, usually walking at a fast pace is safer than running, which can be hard on joints. You could also use a stationary bicycle or swim.

To get the most out of a cardiovascular workout, you should try to reach your target heart rate and maintain it for fifteen to thirty minutes at each session. The target heart rate is the heart rate that provides cardiovascular benefits and is based primarily on your age. To determine your target heart rate, first calculate your maximal heart rate by subtracting your age from 220. Then, multiply that number by 0.70, or 70 percent of your maximal rate. So, if you are fifty years old, your maximal rate would be 170, and your target rate 119. Your heart should beat 119 times per minute when you're at your target heart rate.

Keep in mind that attaining your target heart rate should not be your initial goal, if you're just starting to engage in aerobic activities. You should also never try to work out at your maximal heart rate. Instead, you should slowly build up the time you spend on your cardiovascular workouts.

NIAMS suggests that people who have arthritis should do some form of cardiovascular exercise three times a week, for twenty to thirty minutes a day. If it helps, the exercise can be broken down into ten-minute increments throughout the day. Good examples of cardiovascular exercise for RA patients include riding a stationary bicycle, walking, swimming, and, possibly, low-impact aerobics.

STARTING AN EXERCISE PROGRAM

Once you've made the decision to include physical activity in your daily treatment, talk it over with your physician. He may caution you to avoid doing too much too soon and probably will refer you to a qualified physical therapist who can devise a custom plan for you. Your exercise plan should take into account the severity of your disease, how well you're currently functioning, your lifestyle, and your goals. For instance, if you need to lose weight, you may need a more rigorous exercise program to burn more calories and build muscle (which improves your metabolism). If you're suffering from inflammation, you may be advised to take it more slowly than if you weren't. The key is to follow a program designed just for you.

When you finally do set out to exercise, be sure to take precautions and start slowly. It's best to exercise when you feel the most rested and have the least pain.

Preparing for Exercise

Ready to start exercising? Here's how to get started:

- Always wear appropriate clothing. If you normally wear orthotics or special shoes, make sure you use those when exercising. Avoid clothing that can get in the way of your movements.
- Apply heat to sore joints. Good sources of heat include a hot water bottle, a heating pad, or a hot moist towel. If possible, take a warm shower or whirlpool bath beforehand. Keep the heat mild, not hot, to avoid burns.
- If your joints are inflamed and swollen, apply something cold to them. Wrap a gel pack in a thin towel and place it on the inflamed joint. A bag of frozen vegetables or a bag of ice can also work.
- If necessary, take your pain medications before you exercise, timing it so the relief kicks in during your workout.

- Do some warm-up exercises before you start. Gentle stretching and range-of-motion exercises will warm up the muscles and help prevent injury.

During Your Workout

When you finally do get to your exercises, take precautions to prevent injury and pain. Here's how:

- Breathe deeply and regularly. During exercise, your muscles will require more oxygen, so resist the impulse to hold your breath.
- Use the proper technique for each exercise. Do the recommended number of repetitions, and don't overdo it.
- Keep your movements smooth and flowing. Don't jerk or bounce when you move.
- If something you attempt starts to hurt, skip it.
- Anticipate some muscle soreness. It's normal to experience some muscle fatigue when you exercise.

After You Exercise

- Always devote ten minutes to cooling down. Allow your heart rate and breathing to return to normal. Gently stretch your muscles, too. Don't overstretch, and avoid jerky movements.
- If joints hurt after exercising, apply a cold gel pack, a bag of frozen vegetables, or a bag of ice. Whichever option you choose, wrap it in a thin towel. Apply the cold for up to twenty minutes to reduce inflammation.

KNOW WHEN TO STOP

People who have RA should take extra precautions to guard against exercising too strenuously. You should be on the lookout for signs that you're overdoing it, which are:

- Unusual or persistent fatigue
- Pain that lasts longer than an hour
- Decreased range of motion
- Increased joint swelling

If you find you are experiencing these problems after you exercise, consult your physician and/or physical therapist. Chances are, you need to adjust your routine.

STICKING WITH IT

Now that you've decided to incorporate exercise into your life, you want to make it part of your routine. Here are some ways to help ensure you get your share of regular physical activity:

- Choose activities you enjoy. Don't put yourself through a regimen you don't like. If it helps, enlist a friend to exercise with you, or sign up for a class. You might also try adding music to your routine.
- Make sure you start slowly. Launching an overly ambitious exercise program will make you vulnerable to injury, which will quickly put an end to your plans. Instead, start small and work toward larger goals.
- Listen to your body. A nagging ache is telling you to slow down and take it easy. A dizzy spell during aerobic activity is a cue to sit down. Whenever something doesn't feel right, make sure to pay attention, and rest before resuming activity.
- If you abhor exercise, think about ways to become more active in your daily routine. Park far from the entrance to a building. Clean the house more frequently. Carry your own bags of groceries.
- To prevent boredom from setting in, mix up your routine every month or so. Consider asking your physical therapist

for new exercises, or alter the order in which you complete the ones you're doing.

- Set goals. Before you start, come up with some small, attainable goals as well as some long-term, big picture goals. As you attain each goal, you'll achieve a sense of accomplishment, and that's a boon for anyone who wants to make exercise a habit.
- Once you feel strong enough, consider attempting more recreational exercise. Activities like hiking, cross-country skiing, and bicycling will make getting fit more enjoyable.

THE ROLE OF REST

All this talk about exercise doesn't negate the fact that rest still plays a critical role for the patient who has RA. Rest is the only way to ease the inflammation in your joints. Adequate rest also helps combat the fatigue that plagues RA sufferers. In addition, rest is important to your emotional and mental well-being, and your overall health.

For starters, make sure you get enough sleep every night. Most adults need at least eight hours of sleep every night. In patients with RA, those needs might increase to as much as ten hours. But sleep may be difficult to get when you're wracked with aches and pains and coping with the stress of living with a chronic disease. If you suffer from insomnia, talk to your physician. Relaxation techniques like deep breathing, taking the time to learn and practice good sleep habits, or an occasional sleep remedy might be necessary to induce a good night's sleep.

During the day, you may need to pause from your routine to take a brief nap. A ten- to twenty-minute nap may be all that's needed to restore your waning energy. If that's not possible, look for ways to adjust your routine, so that you alternate between rest and activity. The goal should be to limit your bouts of fatigue, so that you don't become overtired.

When you're experiencing a flare-up, make sure you tip the balance of activity in favor of resting, even using splints, if necessary, to protect your joints from stress. Once the flare-up diminishes, try to get more exercise, so that you can maintain your flexibility, strength, and endurance. Remember, it's a well-balanced regimen of both rest and exercise that will help control the symptoms of RA.

PROFILE

CAROLYN

In the beginning, Carolyn thought for sure that she had carpal tunnel syndrome. Her job as an advertising saleswoman kept her on the computer constantly—and "eating" Advil all the time, too.

Her mother, a nurse, convinced her to see a doctor. "The only reason I went was so my mother would quit bugging me," Carolyn says. Much to her surprise, the doctor, who happened to be a rheumatologist, immediately took some X-rays, sent her blood to a lab, and did a complete evaluation. "Here all I kept saying was that my hands hurt, and he told me to get undressed," she says. "It was really rather unnerving. It wasn't until later on that I learned he was doing a complete evaluation."

When she went to see him for a diagnosis, she was told she had overlapping autoimmune diseases—rheumatoid arthritis, Sjögren's syndrome, and lupus. Carolyn was devastated. She had no idea what the words even meant, but she knew the diagnosis was dire because the doctor looked so sad when he broke the news. His expression created fear, and Carolyn began to wonder if she was going to wind up in a wheelchair or if she'd be around for her kids, who were then five and nine.

Carolyn took copious notes of what her doctor said, then began doing her own intensive research. The doctor put her on Plaquenil, ibuprofen, and a sleep medication. Soon she was overwhelmed with fatigue as the RA took over.

"I was totally unprepared for the fatigue," she says. "It was like the first trimester of pregnancy, compounded by all the body aches. In the morning, you feel really, really stiff. You feel like a truck ran over you. It was really overwhelming."

A high-energy working mother of two, Carolyn, who was thirty-seven at the time she was diagnosed, resisted what her body craved: a carefully balanced mix of rest and exercise. Her children were still young, and she traveled a lot for work. And though she loved bicycling and gardening, she was finding it hard to make time to exercise. Friends finally convinced her to join them on early morning walks around a track. She became a committed walker who was out there even when the wind chills were well below zero. Carolyn loved it, but foot surgery for a bunion put an end to that routine.

When her friends suggested she try an early morning Pilates class, Carolyn decided to give it a shot. These days, she's up at 5:30 a.m. every morning to get to her class. She says it's the best thing she ever did. She feels more limber and flexible and has more strength.

"It took me a long time to realize how much exercise helps," says Carolyn, now forty-seven. "It took me five years to realize that I need to rest. I've had to learn to work with my disease, not against it."

For four years, she carried a page from a calendar in her purse that read "respect your fatigue" as a constant reminder to stop and rest. When she travels now, Carolyn will sleep on the plane. She'll also make the effort to sit and relax. At hotels, she makes time to do her exercises.

Fortunately, she's had no symptoms of lupus, and she's vigilant about symptoms of Sjögren's. She drinks a lot of water to maintain the moisture in her eyes and mouth, and makes sure to see a dentist for regular checkups to reduce the bacterial growth that the dryness can cause.

Meanwhile, her RA comes and goes. A rise in barometric pressure, a stressful day at work, or a sleepless night are all triggers that can worsen her arthritis pain. Even eating poorly can make her tired. But most days, she says, she feels good. She continues to take her Pilates class two or three times a week, and to pay attention to her body's need for rest.

"I think I've been really lucky," Carolyn says. "But I work hard on staying well. To me, you have to be proactive, not reactive. You have to take control of this disease and manage it, not let RA control you."

CHAPTER SEVEN ❧

Achieving Pain Relief

Treating RA involves a two-pronged approach: First, you want to relieve the pain, and second, you want to halt the progression of the disease. We'll start by taking a look at the way your physician might try to help alleviate your aches, pain, and inflammation through the use of nonsteroidal anti-inflammatory drugs, which include aspirin, traditional NSAIDs (pronounced "en-saids" and including Aleve and Motrin), and COX-2 inhibitors (Celebrex), or corticosteroids. Slowing the progression of RA involves other medications called disease-modifying antirheumatic drugs, or DMARDs, and biologic agents, which will be discussed in the next chapter.

ASPIRIN: THE FIRST ANALGESIC

As long ago as the fifth century BC, Hippocrates, considered the father of modern medicine, was said to have used the ground-up bark of willow trees to treat people who were suffering from aches and pains. Willow bark contains salicin, the pain ingredient in a class of medications known as salicylates.

By the late 1800s, salicylates had become the standard drug for the treatment of arthritis. But the treatment was very poorly tolerated and irritating to the stomach. A young German chemist named Felix Hoffmann, who was working for Bayer, set out to develop a treatment that would help his father, who suffered from RA. In 1897, he succeeded when he synthesized acetylsalicylic acid (ASA). Modern aspirin was born.

Today, aspirin is one of the world's safest and least expensive pain relievers, with more than 100 years of proven and effective treatment for a variety of ailments. It is the active ingredient in more than fifty over-the-counter medications. Recent research suggests that it may have healing powers well beyond pain relief; it may also protect patients from an array of conditions including heart disease, Alzheimer's, stroke, and certain cancers.

While aspirin was once widely used in the treatment of RA pain, its use today has been virtually replaced by other anti-inflammatories that can be taken in smaller doses with the same beneficial effects. In the past, high-dose aspirin therapy typically involved taking twenty to thirty regular-strength aspirin tablets a day and had to be prescribed under the close supervision of a physician, with regular monitoring of blood salicylate levels. Too much aspirin caused bleeding in the stomach and ringing in the ears, a condition known as tinnitus.

Side Effects of Aspirin

The most common side effect of aspirin is stomach upset. Some patients may experience increased bleeding, a ringing in their ears, nausea, indigestion, or heartburn. Some people may also pass small amounts of blood in their stools, a problem that can lead to anemia, a deficiency in red blood cells. More serious side effects include gastritis, stomach ulcers, bleeding ulcers, and liver abnormalities.

Before taking any over-the-counter medication, talk to your doctor. Although aspirin is safe with many prescription drugs, it may produce side effects with others. You should also tell your doctor about any history of allergies to aspirin and any problems with asthma, stomach ulcers, and bleeding, as well as kidney or liver problems.

NSAIDS

Most doctors today treat RA pain with an NSAID. These medications offer a viable alternative to aspirin, and in some patients produce less stomach upset. More than twenty million Americans regularly use an NSAID. While many of these medications are sold over the counter, other stronger varieties are often available only by prescription.

The first of the modern NSAIDs, indomethacin, made its market debut in 1956. Other NSAIDs soon followed. The most popular ones include ibuprofen (Advil, Motrin, and Nuprin) and naproxen (Aleve), but there are actually many other ones available, both in over-the-counter and stronger prescription forms.

Then in 1999, another category of NSAIDs was introduced, the COX-2 inhibitors. These new anti-inflammatory remedies were said to be gentler on the stomach and gave patients another option for pain relief. The market for these products boomed. Today, these COX-2 inhibitors are a multibillion-dollar industry.

How NSAIDs Work

All NSAIDs essentially do the same thing: They reduce fever and inflammation and bring about pain relief. Unlike steroids, which reduce inflammation by mimicking natural hormones produced by the body, NSAIDs contain no steroids, hence the name. Instead, NSAIDs work by interfering with the body's production of prostaglandins, proteins that perform several functions in the body, but that also cause pain and inflammation.

NSAIDs inhibit prostaglandins by blocking an enzyme involved in their production called cyclooxygenase, or COX. These enzymes come in at least two forms: COX-1 aids in the production of helpful prostaglandins that perform tasks like protecting the lining of the stomach, helping blood to clot, and regulating the flow of blood to the kidneys. COX-2, on the other hand, is involved in making the prostaglandins that cause pain. The problem is, traditional NSAIDs were nonselective and blocked both COX-1 and COX-2 enzymes.

Not only do the traditional NSAIDs block COX-2 enzymes, but they also inhibit some COX-1 enzymes as well. So at the same time that these NSAIDs help alleviate pain and swelling, they also cause gastrointestinal problems, such as ulcers and bleeding. The newer class of NSAIDs, the selective COX-2 inhibitors, block only COX-2, which suggests they are less damaging to the stomach. And unlike aspirin and traditional NSAIDs, COX-2 inhibitors do not inhibit the clotting of blood.

The Traditional NSAIDs

For a long time, aspirin remained the only analgesic for pain relief. But in patients with RA, the high dosages required to achieve pain relief made aspirin a less than perfect option. The debut of indomethacin and the subsequent NSAIDs gave people another choice. Today, there are about twenty types of NSAIDs available, both in over-the-counter and stronger prescription forms.

Below is a list of traditional NSAIDs:

- Diclofenac (Voltaren or Voltaren XR)
- Diclofenac/misoprostol (Arthrotec)
- Diflunisal (Dolobid)
- Etodolac (Lodine)
- Fenoprofen (Nalfon)
- Flurbiprofen (Ansaid)
- Ibuprofen (Advil, Motrin, Nuprin, Medipren)

- Indomethacin (Indocin)
- Ketoprofen (Orudis, Orudis KT, Actron)
- Magnesium choline trisalicylate (Trilisate)
- Meclofenamate (Meclomen)
- Meloxicam (Mobic)
- Nabumetone (Relafen)
- Naproxen (Naprosyn)
- Naproxen sodium (Naprelan, Anaprox, Anaprox DS, Aleve, Naprosyn)
- Oxaprozin (Daypro)
- Piroxicam (Feldene)
- Salsalate (Disalcid)
- Sulindac (Clinoril)

Before taking a traditional NSAID, let your doctor know of any allergies to aspirin or other anti-inflammatory medications. You should also let him know if you've had asthma, nasal polyps, stomach ulcers, bleeding problems, colitis, high blood pressure, or kidney and liver problems. In addition, be sure to tell your doctor about other medications you are taking, including vitamins and supplements.

The New NSAIDs
In 1999, a new category of NSAIDs was introduced, one that promised fewer side effects with the same benefits as the traditional versions. These were the COX-2 inhibitors, named for the enzyme that these new NSAIDs inhibited. The FDA-approved COX-2 inhibitor is Celecoxib (Celebrex). (Please refer to A Note to Readers page vii.)

Before you start taking a COX-2 inhibitor, be sure to alert your doctor to any previous allergies to aspirin or other anti-inflammatory medications. Tell your doctor about other medications you are taking, including vitamins and supplements. You should also tell him if you've had high blood pressure, fluid retention, swelling, asthma, nasal polyps, stomach ulcer, colitis, or kidney or liver problems.

In addition, he should know about prior heart attacks, stroke, or blood clots. Studies have suggested that rofecoxib (Vioxx), once the top-selling COX-2 inhibitor, was associated with a higher risk for heart disease. The risks were significant enough that Merck, the company that distributed Vioxx, took it off the market.

Side Effects of NSAIDs

There's no doubt that NSAIDs are highly effective in relieving pain from RA. But these medications can cause disturbing side effects, especially if they're taken for a long time or in high doses. As many as 100,000 people each year are hospitalized for gastrointestinal problems related to the ingestion of NSAIDs. Approximately 16,500 die of these problems.

Though the COX-2 inhibitors generally cause less gastrointestinal distress, all NSAIDs, including aspirin, can produce stomach upset. Symptoms may include nausea, abdominal pain or cramps, diarrhea, constipation, gas, and indigestion. Some patients also complain of headaches, drowsiness, difficulty concentrating, and rash. In more serious cases, NSAIDs can cause bleeding and ulcers in the lining of your stomach. Taking your NSAID with food or a glass of milk can help reduce gastrointestinal upset.

In rare cases, NSAIDs have been associated with problems in the liver and kidneys, which require discontinuing use of the drug. Some patients may experience prolonged bleeding and bruising; NSAIDs can also cause fluid retention in some people.

Some drugs can exacerbate the side effects of NSAIDs, which will increase your risk for bleeding and ulcers. For instance, you should be careful when combining NSAIDs with alendrondonate (Fosamax) and risedronate (Actonel), which are used to treat osteoporosis, and corticosteroids such as prednisone, which may be used to treat RA. Anticoagulants such as warfarin, which is used to prevent blood clotting, should also not be taken with NSAIDs, since both medications slow clotting and can cause bleeding. While COX-2 inhibitors may be safer to use with warfarin, they should also be used with caution because the combination can increase the risk for bleeding.

Countering Side Effects

Taking your NSAIDs with food or a glass of milk can help ease the problems of GI distress. Some people may also need to take medication to protect their stomachs. For instance, misoprostol (Cytotec) may be prescribed to prevent stomach irritation. Arthrotec is one drug that may help you avoid stomach distress since it combines misoprostol (Cytotec) and diclofenac (Voltaren). You may also be given a proton pump inhibitor such as lansoprazole (Prevacid) to help your stomach reduce acid production and prevent gastrointestinal complications. Antacids may also be used for that purpose.

Once you do start taking an NSAID, be on the lookout for possible side effects. If they do arise, immediately discuss them with your doctor. Serious ones like persistent indigestion or nausea, and dark-colored bowel movements, warrant immediate attention. Remember, different people respond differently to different NSAIDs. Simply trying a different kind might help relieve the side effects.

Are You at Risk for Side Effects?

Fortunately, not everyone will experience side effects from the use of NSAIDs. And not everyone will experience them severely. Certain populations are at greater risk than others. You are at greater risk if you:

- Are age sixty or older
- Had stomach ulcers in the past
- Take warfarin (Coumadin)
- Take prednisone
- Are getting chemotherapy
- Use tobacco
- Drink three or more alcoholic beverages a day
- Have been taking an NSAID for a long time
- Take high doses of your NSAID
- Take more than one NSAID
- Are in poor overall health

Which One Is Right for You?

With so many NSAIDs to choose from, you will need to work with your doctor to choose the best drug. Among the factors he'll take into consideration are the side effects of each drug, your risk factors, how often you'll need to take the drug, the cost, and your preferences. Some NSAIDs are taken several times a day, while others are taken just once or twice.

The cost of the drugs varies greatly, too. Some traditional NSAIDs are available as generics and can cost as little as fifteen dollars a month. The COX-2 inhibitors do not come in generic form and can cost more than seventy-five dollars a month.

CORTICOSTEROIDS: TAMING THE INFLAMMATION

When corticosteroids, also called glucocorticoids, first emerged on the market in the 1940s, they were touted as a cure for RA. In fact, the effects of high-dose corticosteroids on RA were so dramatic that Dr. Phillip Hench and his colleague Edward Kendall received the Nobel Prize for their work in 1950.

But the relief came at a high and terrible price: Corticosteroids, or simply steroids, caused serious side effects, especially at these high doses. The drugs caused weight gain, increased appetite, water retention, acne, facial hair growth, nervousness, insomnia, depression, and nausea. In the long run, steroids could cause osteoporosis, menstrual irregularities, muscle weakness, cataracts, infection, and glaucoma. If you had diabetes, steroids could worsen your symptoms. They also caused patients to have a full, round face (known as a moon face) and made them more likely to bruise. Clearly, steroids were not the perfect answer.

For a while, physicians steered clear of prescribing steroids. Today, steroids are being used again to treat RA and numerous other conditions, but with much greater caution and control. The drugs are used when a patient's arthritis cannot be controlled by NSAIDs and DMARDs or when a patient cannot take these medications because of side effects. Steroids are now given in the smallest dose possible and, often, for a temporary period. Typically, they are prescribed for what is called bridge therapy—to control inflammation while waiting for slow-acting DMARDs to take effect. Once the inflammation is reduced, the patient is slowly weaned off the steroid. In some patients, steroids are injected into joints to help reduce swelling, warmth, and pain for up to six weeks.

Besides reducing inflammation, steroids can alleviate pain. But the disappearance of your pain is just that—temporary relief from the pain. The good news is that there is now some evidence that steroids may actually slow the rate of joint damage.

OTHER SOURCES OF PAIN RELIEF

In some cases, NSAIDs may not work. If your pain is severe, your doctor may prescribe a non-opioid analgesic like tramadol (Ultram) or an opioid, or a narcotic analgesic such as oxycodone (OxyContin, Roxicodone). If oral remedies fail to provide pain relief, your doctor may prescribe topical analgesics. These drugs come in the form of creams, salves, and ointments that can be rubbed over

the site of the pain without any systemic side effects. The active ingredients in these remedies vary and include capsaicin, a natural
substance found in cayenne peppers; salicylates, the same active ingredient in aspirin; and various counterirritants such as menthol,
camphor, eucalyptus oil, and oil of wintergreen.

THE IMPORTANCE OF MINIMIZING YOUR PAIN

You may pride yourself on having a high threshold for pain, and
maybe it was helpful in the past when you hit your thumb with a
hammer or stubbed your toe on furniture. But living day-to-day with
the excruciating pain caused by RA can be not only physically drain-
ing but mentally and emotionally frustrating. Being able to control
your pain is critical to your quality of life and emotional well-being.

That said, start by taking the lowest dose of medication possible to reduce your pain, and then gradually increase the dosage if
necessary. Never take more than your prescribed dosage since that
will enhance the likelihood for side effects. And make sure to tell
your doctor about any problems, side effects, and concerns.

PROFILE

SUSAN

Susan was a very healthy, active forty-three-year-old woman and mother of three. She was working part-time and studying toward her master's degree when she started developing symptoms of rheumatoid arthritis. At the time, she was repairing her own VW, painting and wallpapering her house, tending a vegetable garden, and building a room in her attic.

The symptoms developed from out of nowhere. For a few days, she couldn't lift her arm. On other days, she couldn't get in a car without lifting her right leg using her hands. Then her hands began to swell, and she started awakening with morning stiffness.

Susan endured these intermittent symptoms for six months before finally speaking to a friend who was a doctor. Her friend immediately suspected she had RA and gave her the name of a rheumatologist.

Blood tests confirmed what her friend suspected—Susan had RA. "My rheumatologist said my rheumatoid factor was so high I would probably end up in a wheelchair," Susan recalls. "In my mind I'd turned into a five-year-old, and I remember responding immediately, 'No, I won't!' or as my kids used to say, with a stamp of the foot, 'No, I not!'"

In the years that followed, Susan began to view her life as a series of games. There was the game of finding the right doctor, the game of determining the correct mix of medications, the game of finding helpful alternative treatments, the game of pain management, and the game of forging a strong partnership with her doctor.

Managing her pain was especially challenging. "I'm not particularly interested in stopping the progression of the disease," she says. "I actually don't think I mind having RA—I don't see it as an enemy, and I don't fight it exactly. It's mine and it's there to be solved. It is the pain I wish not to have."

To rein in the pain, she began by taking sixteen aspirins a day. But the heavy dosage made her ears ring. She also tried Plaquenil, to no avail. Then she tried various NSAIDs. Each drug met with limited, short-term success.

"There always seemed to be another one until there weren't any anymore," she says.

Susan also tried gold injections for a time and had cortisone when the pain got severe. She is now taking Plaquenil, Arava, and six Tylenol a day. "This is the right mix for now," Susan says. "The mix works for a year, year and a half or two years, then does not. And the search for a new mix begins. That's why one needs a good doctor to partner with. I've been working on my medication regimen for twenty-five years."

Meanwhile, she did yoga and tried weight lifting. She also bought a waterbed and slept a lot. She tried various diets and vitamins and minerals, stopped eating plants like tomatoes and eggplant, and became a vegetarian.

She continued pursuing her master's degree, got involved in a love affair, and moved back to New York City. She also continued working and became proficient in both the MAC and the PC. "I refused to stop or give up," she says. "I accepted my limitations, but I kept heading off in new directions."

When the pain got bad, Susan liked to do a mental technique she called "leaving her body." It was a form of detachment, a way of shifting her attention elsewhere, so she could become numb to the pain. "I would get very silent and think about favorite people and happy incidents," Susan says. "Or I'd turn my attention elsewhere to things I could do, like wallpapering and painting. It would be as if I weren't there."

Susan also tried to reason with her condition. At one point, she decided that RA was the result of her "protective cover," or body armor. As an adult child of alcoholics, she thought she was carrying too much emotional baggage. Having RA, she believed, was the result of holding herself too tightly. "After much therapy, I went to a self-help group that specialized in adult children of alcoholics, where I learned to have my emotions and express them," she says.

At another point, she drowned out her pain by listening to music through headphones. "When the sound feels like it's in the middle of my head, I feel no pain," she explains.

No matter what approach she tried, Susan always found herself in the middle of the pain game. The problem, she said, was the unpredictability of both the disease and the medications she took.

To help her through, she surrounded herself with positive, sympathetic, and empathic people. She needed people who could understand her limitations and could accept that some days, she simply couldn't do what they wanted.

"One of the most important support persons I had is no longer living," Susan recalls. "She died many years ago after a thirteen-year battle with cancer. I spent a lot of time with her going through the dying process, which turned out to be a lesson in living. When I think of how I cope with RA—living despite pain, enjoying the moment, learning and trying new things, traveling to far places, exploring alternatives, being 'open' and receptive—I hear and feel my old friend. She is with me and encourages me."

Over the years, Susan has learned to steer clear of people who complain and talk about illness all the time. "I find it depressing and debilitating," Susan says simply. "I don't like to think of myself as judgmental, but I try to be self-protective. There's a certain kind of person who responds 'softly' when I say I'm having a flare-up. They are sympathetic and empathic, but not jarringly so. I can't describe it exactly except to say they are sensitive and gentle and accepting. They're not trying to make it better because they can't stand that I am in pain."

She also found a rheumatologist who was willing to approach her health care from a team perspective, someone who didn't talk down to her, lent a sympathetic ear when needed, and gave her the reassurance she so often craved. "I needed a doctor who is willing to say, 'How are you today? Let's try this. What do you think?' Most of all, I wanted a doctor who actually wants to take care of me."

CHAPTER EIGHT ✒

Halting the Disease

Not long ago, RA was treated rather conservatively. When a patient was first diagnosed, doctors typically chose the safest medication, usually aspirin or a nonsteroidal anti-inflammatory drug (NSAID). They also urged patients to rest, and maybe try some physical therapy. It wasn't until the disease began to damage the joints that doctors began prescribing more aggressive medications such as the disease-modifying antirheumatic drugs (DMARDs) and biologic response modifiers.

These days, the approach has been reversed and is considerably more aggressive. Researchers began to realize that most of the joint damage in RA typically occurs in the early stages of disease, even before the damage could be seen on X-rays. By halting the damage early on with aggressive treatments, patients were able to enjoy better long-term outcomes and slow, or even prevent, the joint damage that so often occurs with RA. So rather than waiting for the damage to appear on X-rays, doctors are now attempting to slow the destruction early on with the use of DMARDs or another category of medications, called biologic response modifiers or biologic agents.

As the understanding of RA has grown, the number of medications available to treat the disease has escalated. Patients today have multiple options, so that if one medication doesn't work or produces too many side effects, there are others to try. The key is to choose the one that works best for you.

AIMING FOR REMISSION

The ultimate goal of treatment with DMARDs is to get the disease into remission. According to the American College of Rheumatology (ACR), remission is defined as the absence of six factors: symptoms of active inflammatory joint pain; morning stiffness; fatigue; synovitis upon examination of the joints; evidence of progressive damage as seen on sequential X-rays; and elevated levels of erythrocyte sedimentation rate (ESR) or C-reactive protein (CRP) levels.

Sometimes, a single drug is all that is needed to induce a remission. But often patients may need a combination of two or three drugs. In the mid 1990s, researchers in Finland compared patients who received only one DMARD against those who received three. They found that after two years, only 18 percent of those in the group treated with one DMARD went into remission, compared with 40 percent in the group treated with three. Approximately 14 percent of RA patients achieve spontaneous remission, which is a remission induced without drug intervention.

In a follow-up study, some patients in the group that used just one DMARD opted to increase the number of DMARDs in their regimen. But even with the additional medications, the rate of remission was lower than in the group that initially used three DMARDs, suggesting that patients have only "a window of opportunity" in which to take an aggressive approach to treatment. The group that used three DMARDs also had less joint damage and reported less swelling, pain, and loss of mobility.

Unfortunately, not all patients will go into remission, despite the most intensive efforts to find the right treatment regimen. For these patients, the ACR says, the goals are to control disease activity, alleviate the aches and pain, maintain daily functioning, and maximize the patient's quality of life. These goals may be achieved through a combination of NSAIDs, DMARDs, biologics, glucocorticoids, rehabilitation therapy, and analgesics.

WHAT YOU WILL TAKE

Just as the disease is different in every patient, so too is each patient's medication regimen. Usually, what a doctor decides to prescribe depends on your prognosis. In general, younger patients with swelling in more than twenty joints and high levels of rheumatoid factor and elevated ESR levels have a worse prognosis. Patients who have other health problems associated with RA also have a poorer prognosis. These conditions include rheumatoid nodules, Sjögren's syndrome, scleritis, pericardial involvement, inflammation of the blood vessels, and Felty's syndrome, a rare condition that causes an enlarged spleen and a decreased white blood cell count.

Ideally, the patient should be involved in determining the treatment regimen. While it's your doctor's job to present your options, it's your job to share critical information, such as your ability to afford certain medications, your personal preferences, any drug allergies, and preexisting conditions. And it always helps if you're already familiar with the medications that are available for the treatment of RA. These drug classifications include the following:

DMARDs

It's safe to say that virtually all patients with RA will receive treatments with disease-modifying antirheumatic drugs. These slow-acting medications have the potential to hasten the course of RA, thereby preserving joint function; reducing, or even preventing, joint damage; and possibly inducing a remission. For many patients, these drugs enable them to remain fully functional.

Once a patient is diagnosed with RA, treatment with a DMARD should not be delayed more than three months. The choice of treatment and the numbers of DMARDs involved will vary, depending on, among other factors, the severity of the disease and the safety and convenience of administering the drug. Some DMARDs are immunosuppressants, which reduce the functioning of the immune system. Here are the eleven DMARDs commonly used to treat RA:

Methotrexate

A well-established record in the treatment of RA has made methotrexate (Rheumatrex, Trexall) the first drug of choice by rheumatologists treating RA. Initially used to treat people with leukemia, it is also used in high doses as an anti-cancer medication.

Methotrexate, which is an immunosuppressant, is popular for several reasons: The drug is highly effective. It also works faster than other DMARDs, with notable improvements evident in as little as two to three weeks. In addition, methotrexate is convenient; patients need to take the pills all in one day, once a week, or receive a weekly injection. Methotrexate is available in generic form, making it more affordable as well.

More than half of patients using methotrexate stay on it beyond three years. When they do stop, it's usually due to side effects rather than the drug's lack of efficacy. Side effects of methotrexate include nausea, vomiting, and diarrhea. Rare but more serious side effects include inflammation of the lung and lowered blood counts. Long-term use can cause scarring and inflammation of the liver. Studies suggest that taking folic acid or folinic acid can reduce the side effects of methotrexate.

Patients on methotrexate should have their liver function carefully monitored. Alcohol is strictly prohibited. Women in their childbearing years should avoid becoming pregnant since methotrexate can cause fetal death and birth defects. And if you do plan to have children, you should talk to your doctor first (whether you're a man or a woman). Both men and women are generally advised to wait several months after discontinuing methotrexate before trying to conceive.

Hydroxychloroquine

Another popular DMARD in the treatment of RA is hydroxychloroquine (Plaquenil). An anti-malarial medication derived from quinine, HCQ was first used to treat RA in the 1950s. The drug is generally well-tolerated, and improvements typically take a month to six months. HCQ is available in generic form.

Side effects of HCQ are few, though in some patients it can cause nausea, decreased appetite, diarrhea, and rash. These problems are usually resolved by taking the medication with food or adjusting the dosage.

The main risk of any anti-malarial medication is retinopathy. Long-term use of HCQ can cause changes in the retina, though the risk in RA patients is low because of the small dosages typically prescribed. Routine eye exams with an ophthalmologist are important if you're taking HCQ. You should also not take it if you're pregnant or nursing.

Sulfasalazine

Though it was first used to treat RA in the 1930s and 1940s, sulfasalazine did not receive official approval from the U.S. Food and Drug Administration (FDA) until 1996. The drug is considered a well-tolerated treatment for RA that produces improvements in as little as a month. It's also available in generic form.

The predominant side effect of sulfasalazine is stomach upset. Although the medication is most effective when it's taken on an empty stomach, taking it with food can sometimes help relieve gastrointestinal pain. It can also help to start at a low dose and gradually work up to higher dosages. Other side effects, which are rare, include headaches, lowered sperm count—which can be reversed by discontinuing the medication—liver toxicity, and a decrease in blood platelets and white- and red-blood cell-count.

Routine monitoring of the blood, liver, and urine may be done when you're on this medication. This drug should be avoided during pregnancy. People who have an allergy to sulfa should not take sulfasalazine.

Leflunomide

For patients who cannot tolerate methotrexate, leflunomide (Arava) has emerged as a good, equally effective alternative. Leflunomide went on the market in 1998 and was specifically developed for the treatment of RA. The drug is an immune system modifier and works by shutting down the lymphocytes that promote RA. Studies show it relieves pain and swelling, improves functioning, and slows the disease. There is no generic version available.

The benefits of leflunomide kick in around four weeks. The most common side effects involve the gastrointestinal tract, namely diarrhea, nausea, vomiting, and abdominal pain. Some patients may experience hair loss, rash, and elevated liver enzymes. While you're taking leflunomide, it's common for your doctor to routinely monitor your blood and liver.

Leflunomide cannot be taken by pregnant women since the drug does increase the risk for birth defects. Women in their childbearing years should be using reliable birth control if they are prescribed leflunomide.

Blood levels of leflunomide linger after use of this drug, possibly for as long as two years. If you wish to become pregnant after taking leflunomide, you will need to undergo a drug elimination protocol that involves taking an eleven-day course of cholestyramine, a drug that removes bile acids from your body.

Azathioprine (Imuran)

Azathioprine is rarely used in the treatment of RA. As the first immunosuppressant to receive FDA approval for the treatment of RA, azathioprine is used to prevent rejection in patients who have received organ transplants. It is also used as a cancer drug. It is generally not the first drug prescribed for the treatment of RA, but one that doctors turn to after other DMARDs have failed to produce results. Azathioprine is often used in combination therapies. It is available in generic form.

Azathioprine can cause a decrease in the number of blood cells in your bone marrow. Signs of problems include unusual bleeding or bruising, extreme fatigue, pale skin, headache, confusion, dizziness, fast heartbeat, weakness, shortness of breath, and symptoms resembling the flu. It can also cause upset stomach, vomiting, and diarrhea. Because azathioprine is an immunosuppressant, patients on it are at higher risk for infections due to a reduction in white blood cells. In very rare cases, the drug may cause cancer after prolonged use. Tests to monitor blood counts and liver function are performed routinely while a patient is on azathioprine.

Azathioprine should not be used during pregnancy since it can affect the fetal immune system. It may also be temporarily discontinued if you develop an infection.

Gold, Injectable

Originally used to treat tuberculosis, gold injections became a treatment for RA in the 1920s, were used less frequently during the 1930s and early 1940s, and then enjoyed a resurgence in the late

1940s. Gold, whether injected or taken orally, appears to work by interfering with the production of proteins and antibodies in the immune system. Injections of gold are administered in the buttock muscle weekly or monthly, with dosages increased slowly. Improvements are achieved in as little as six weeks or as long as six months. Also called gold sodium, injectable gold is available as thiomalate (Myochrysine) or aurothioglucose (Solganal).

Some patients may experience temporary joint pain shortly after the injections. They may also experience flushing, dizziness, sweating, headache, or blurred vision. Approximately a third of all patients receiving gold injections will experience other side effects, the most common being protein in the urine. Some patients may experience a rash or itching, mouth sores, a metallic taste, or hair loss. More serious but less common side effects include a reduction in blood platelets that causes a decrease in the levels of red and white blood cells and problems with the liver or kidneys.

Patients receiving injections of gold will have their blood, liver, and kidneys routinely monitored. Women who wish to become pregnant are advised to discontinue gold injections several months before conceiving.

Gold, Oral

The oral form of gold is considered to be one of the less effective treatments for RA and is rarely used today. It's also more likely to be used for patients with mild cases. Improvements generally take six weeks to six months. Oral gold is not available in generic form and is sold as auranofin (Ridaura). The pill is taken once or twice a day.

Although generally regarded as being less effective than injectable gold, oral gold does produce fewer serious side effects. The most common are cramping, diarrhea, decreased appetite, flatulence, and heartburn. Some patients may also experience nausea, rash, itching, and mouth sores. In rare cases, oral gold may cause hair loss, a metallic taste, hives, and problems in the blood.

During treatment, your physician will monitor your blood counts and urine. Women who wish to become pregnant are advised to discontinue gold before conceiving.

Cyclosporine

Although sometimes prescribed as a single therapy, cyclosporine (Neoral) is usually given in combination with methotrexate when methotrexate alone has failed. An immune suppressant, cyclosporine has been prescribed primarily for people who have had organ transplants as a way to keep the immune system from rejecting the new organ. The drug is rarely used to treat RA.

Side effects of cyclosporine include high blood pressure and reduction in kidney function. Patients may also experience tremors, headaches, dizziness, rash, nausea, diarrhea, stomach upset, and increased growth of body hair.

Patients on cyclosporine are closely monitored for high blood pressure and given frequent kidney function tests. Sometimes they must discontinue use of the drug if their blood pressure goes up or the levels of creatinine in their kidneys are elevated. Patients are closely checked for infections. Though there are no studies on the effects of cyclosporine in pregnancy, women are generally advised to discontinue the drug if they conceive.

Penicillamine

Penicillamine (Cuprimine, Depen) is rarely used to treat RA today. It works by decreasing the formation of antibodies, reducing the function of T cells, and helping to eliminate damaging molecules called free radicals. Although quite effective, penicillamine has been replaced by some of the safer DMARDs that produce fewer side effects. As many as 40 percent of all patients abandon use of penicillamine in the first year because of its side effects. And because of these side effects, the dose of penicillamine is increased slowly, so that improvements aren't seen for as long as two to nine months.

The most problematic side effect is a reduction in platelet counts, which causes a decline in red blood cells as well as immune-boosting white blood cells. The lowered blood counts render the patient vulnerable to infections. Other side effects include rash, upset stomach, nausea, vomiting, diarrhea, and a change in taste. Some patients also experience mouth sores. Rare but more serious side effects include protein in the urine, kidney problems, the development of autoimmune conditions, and muscle weakness.

Routine blood counts and urine tests are usually conducted while a patient is taking penicillamine. Women wishing to become pregnant should avoid penicillamine since it does cause birth defects.

Cyclophosphamide

Patients who have severe or life-threatening forms of RA, possibly involving vital organs, may be candidates for cyclophosphamide (Cytoxan). This powerful immune suppressant is a cancer treatment with severe side effects that restrict its use to the more serious cases of RA. For instance, a patient who develops Felty's syndrome or vasculitis might be put on cyclophosphamide since the benefits may outweigh the risks. If effective, the medication is also fast-acting, with improvements seen in as little as seven to ten days.

Cyclophosphamide is fraught with side effects, including nausea, vomiting, decreased appetite, hair loss, and rash. Like azathioprine, cyclophosphamide can reduce white blood cell count, putting the patient at risk for severe blood problems and infections. The risk increases as the dose goes up. Cyclophosphamide can also cause cystitis, or bladder inflammation, which makes urination uncomfortable and can cause blood in the urine. In the long run, cyclophosphamide may raise the risk for cancers, specifically bladder cancer and blood cancers such as leukemia and lymphomas.

Another disturbing side effect of cyclophosphamide is infertility. In addition, both men and women are advised to use birth control when taking cyclophosphamide since the drug can cause birth defects. Because of the seriousness of these side effects, cyclophosphamide is typically a last alternative.

Minocycline
Some researchers believe that infections may play a role in RA. That theory is buoyed by the fact that minocycline (Minocin), an antibiotic in the tetracycline family, may cause an improvement in the symptoms of RA. Minocycline appears to slow the progression of joint damage and prevent disability in patients who have mild forms of the disease. Exactly how minocycline works on RA is unknown. In addition to its antimicrobial effects, minocycline appears to decrease the production of substances that cause inflammation, including prostaglandins and leukotrienes. At the same time, it increases the production of interleukin-10, a substance in the blood that reduces inflammation.

Compared to other DMARDs, minocycline has few side effects. Some patients may experience dizziness, rash, and stomach problems. In rare cases, patients have described lupus-like reactions to minocycline. Other possible side effects include a change in skin pigmentation, a growth of fungi or yeast, and increased sensitivity to the sun.

Patients on minocycline should not take antacids, calcium, magnesium, or iron since these substances may interfere with the absorption of minocycline. They should also avoid intensive sun exposure and wear sunblock. In addition, women taking minocycline should not get pregnant since it can affect the fetus.

Biologic Response Modifiers

In recent years, the treatment of RA has experienced a major advance with the development of biologic response modifiers (BRMs). These medications are not a manufactured chemical, but rather they are created by living cells and function like substances already found in your body. They focus in particular on the transmission of messages sent between chemical messengers called cytokines.

To understand how biologics work, you need to know about the events that occur within the immune system that bring on RA. Biologic response modifiers interfere with these events.

For reasons that are unclear, something occurs in the body of a person who develops RA that triggers the immune system into action against the body's own cells. Macrophages, key players in the immune reaction, are activated, and in the process release chemicals that lure other white blood cells to the scene of a perceived invasion by an antigen. In doing their job, macrophages produce substantial amounts of cytokines, chemicals that allow components of the immune system to communicate with one another.

Certain cytokines are pro-inflammatory and alert immune system cells to become inflamed. When these cytokines tell immune system cells to promote inflammation, they do it by attaching to a receptor cell, which then complies and starts to release the chemicals leading to inflammation and damage. Two cytokines that deliver the pro-inflammatory message are tumor necrosis factor (TNF) and interleukin-1 (IL-1). In healthy people, small amounts of these cytokines are needed for the proper functioning of the immune system. Their actions are balanced out by anti-inflammatory proteins. But in people who have RA, these pro-inflammatory cytokines occur in such large amounts that the activity is off balance.

Cytokines perpetuate the growth of blood vessels going to the synovium, which, in turn, causes the joint to feel warm.

When cytokines leak into the bloodstream, they bring on the fatigue that is virtually always a part of RA. Cytokines are also responsible for the production of prostaglandins and leukotrienes, substances that promote pain and inflammation.

Three of the BRMs on the market interfere with the pro-inflammatory messages of TNF, and one with IL-1. All of them target the pathways that bring on the joint inflammation and damage associated with RA. By doing so, they reduce inflammation and ease the pain, fatigue, and symptoms of the disease. Here are the four BRMs currently approved for the treatment of RA.

Etanercept (Enbrel)
Introduced in 1998 as the first BRM, etanercept has had a profound effect on the treatment of RA. The drug works by mimicking the action of TNF receptors in the body. Enbrel is a free-floating TNF receptor that intercepts naturally occurring TNF molecules and prevents them from getting to the target receptor cells to deliver their pro-inflammatory message.

Etanercept captures TNF before it can hook up with its receptor. When TNF is attached to etanercept, it cannot communicate its pro-inflammatory message. It is commonly called an anti-TNF drug or TNF blocker.

Etanercept is typically prescribed to patients with moderate to severe RA and who have not responded to DMARDs. It may be given alone or in combination with methotrexate.

The effects of etanercept kick in in as quickly as two weeks. Many patients notice maximum benefits by three months. Studies show it decreases pain, fatigue, and stiffness. It also improves day-to-day functioning.

As a protein, etanercept is injected subcutaneously into the skin. To prevent irritation at the injection site, patients should alternate the injection sites, which may include the abdomen, thigh, and arm. And because it is a protein, etanercept must also be refrigerated.

Side effects of etanercept are few, though some patients experience reactions at the injection site, headaches, and nausea. Patients may also be at risk for infections. In extremely rare cases, etanercept may cause multiple sclerosis, inflammation of the eyes, and blood disorders that could lead to death. Patients who previously had tuberculosis (TB), who have poorly controlled diabetes, who have poorly controlled heart failure, or who are prone to infections may not be good candidates for etanercept. Testing for prior TB exposure is essential before starting this medication.

Infliximab (Remicade)

The introduction of etanercept was followed in 1999 by the debut of infliximab. This drug is a monoclonal antibody that was biogenetically manufactured in a lab—it's part mouse and part human—and works by decreasing the number of pro-inflammatory cytokines. Infliximab works by attaching to the TNF molecule and permanently inactivating it.

Infliximab is administered intravenously during a two-hour outpatient infusion. Patients typically receive three initial infusions, and then need to receive a dosage once every eight weeks. Treatment may take place in a local infusion center, an outpatient clinic at the hospital, the doctor's office, or at home with the aid of a trained nurse.

The infusion process is not difficult. A health-care professional, usually a nurse, will check your blood pressure, pulse rate, and temperature, and then place an IV in your arm. While the medication is delivered to you intravenously, you will be regularly monitored. But you can use this time to read, relax, catch up on work, or listen to music.

Infliximab is administered in combination with methotrexate, and the two together have been found to reduce the symptoms of

RA and slow the progression of joint damage. Patients generally experience an improvement in their physical functioning.

But the drug does have side effects, including itching and stinging at the site of the infusion. Less commonly, patients may experience low blood pressure, rash, fever, achiness, chills, hives, chest pain, or difficulty breathing. By treating the patient beforehand with the allergy antihistamine diphenhydramine (Benadryl) and acetaminophen (Tylenol), some of these side effects may be reduced.

More serious side effects include an increased risk for infection, including tuberculosis, and a possible increased risk for lymphoma. Treatment may also result in the production of auto-antibodies, antibodies that target your body as an infecting agent. In rare cases, a patient may develop lupus-like syndrome. Again, testing for prior TB exposure is needed before taking this medication. Infliximab must be discontinued if serious symptoms emerge.

Adalimumab (Humira)

The newest of the BRMs, adalimumab debuted in 2003. Like infliximab, adalimumab is a monoclonal antibody that combats the pro-inflammatory TNF and renders it ineffective. It is made with human proteins.

Used alone or in combination with DMARDs such as methotrexate, adalimumab can help lessen the symptoms of RA and improve mobility. Patients will notice they are less fatigued and will experience the disease in fewer joints. The improvements may emerge in as soon as two weeks, but full effect of the drug may take up to three months.

Adalimumab is given by self-administered injections every two weeks. To prevent irritation at the injection site, patients should alternate the injection sites, which may include the abdomen, thigh, and arm. And because it is a protein, adalimumab must also be refrigerated.

Side effects for adalimumab are similar to those of etanercept and infliximab, with injection site reactions and an increased risk for infection being of greatest concern. Testing for prior exposure to TB must be done before taking this drug.

Anakinra (Kineret)

Anakinra is a man-made receptor antagonist and the only BRM that acts against IL-1. It was introduced in 2001. The drug works by plugging up the IL-1 receptor, so the IL-1 cannot send the message to promote inflammation, thereby slowing the progression of the disease. Though it is a man-made protein, it is similar to the naturally occurring protein interleukin-1 receptor antagonist. The drug decreases pain and swelling and helps protect the integrity of the joint.

Anakinra may be given alone or in combination with a DMARD, but it cannot be prescribed with other BRMs. The combination of anakinra with another biologic greatly increases the risk for infection. Anakinra also cannot be used in patients with a hypersensitivity to proteins derived from E. coli.

Anakinra is taken daily by injection. Each dose comes in a pre-filled syringe. And because it is a protein, the medication must be kept in a refrigerator.

The most common side effect of anakinra is a reaction at the injection site. Minor redness, bruising, swelling, and pain may occur where the injection is made; these symptoms may last up to a month. If the injection site swells or becomes itchy, you might want to apply a cold pack on the skin before and after injection. And like other BRMs, anakinra may also increase your risk for infection. In rare cases, you may experience a reduction in white blood cell count. As a result of this possibility, your blood count will be closely monitored while you are taking anakinra.

Other Cautions

Biologics are powerful medications that can produce amazing results in patients with RA. But it's important to take these medications under the close supervision of your rheumatologist and to be careful of preexisting conditions that may exacerbate the side effects of these drugs. Patients who have had TB, major infections, multiple sclerosis, congestive heart failure, and lymphoma should discuss these conditions with their doctors before taking a biologic.

These drugs also pose additional risks. You should not get a live vaccine while taking a BRM because your immune system is compromised. In addition, you should avoid these medications if you're considering getting pregnant or nursing. Most of these drugs have not been tested in pregnant women, and most drugs are passed through mother's milk.

Finally, be sure to discuss any concern at all with your doctor before taking these medications or while you're on them. No symptom is too minor to warrant a conversation with your doctor, who can make sure you're taking the right medication at the proper dosage.

Prosorba Column: The One-of-a-Kind Option

Patients with severe RA who have had no improvements with DMARDs or the biologics may be given a treatment called Protein A immunoadsorption using a device called the Prosorba column. The device was approved for the treatment of RA in 1999.

The column itself is a cylinder shaped like a soup can with a filter containing a sandlike substance called Protein A. The procedure works like dialysis and cleanses your blood of the destructive antibodies that cause the damaging effects of RA.

Treatment with the Prosorba column consists of twelve weekly sessions, each lasting about two hours. While you're seated or lying down, a nurse places a needle in each of your arms. Your blood is slowly drawn from one arm and then passed through a machine that separates the blood into blood cells and plasma, which is the liquid portion of your blood. The plasma, which contains the harmful antibodies, is cycled through the Prosorba column, where the antibodies cling to Protein A. Once purified, the clean plasma is rejoined with the blood cells and returned to the vein of the other arm. The clean plasma still contains the antibodies that protect the body against infection.

Like all RA medications, Protein A immunoadsorption may cause side effects. People who use this therapy are at greater risk for infection. During treatment, some people experience a drop in blood pressure, which can be alleviated by giving extra intravenous fluids. In the day or two after treatment, you may notice fatigue or mild flulike symptoms. It may also cause anemia. The treatment is not recommended for patients who take ACE inhibitors for high blood pressure; those who have had heart disease, stroke, or blood clots; and pregnant women.

Improvements may occur in three to four months. Many patients can get months of relief from a single course of therapy, with some getting more than eighteen months of relief. On average, patients get thirty-seven weeks of relief. If severe symptoms return, the twelve-week course of Prosorba column therapy can be repeated as often as necessary.

PROFILE

BRUCE

Since he was fourteen years old, Bruce has suffered from severe allergies. At forty-two, he developed asthma. Then at fifty-nine, he was diagnosed with RA. He blames it all on a faulty immune system that has a penchant for attacking his own body.

Bruce says he can't be sure exactly when he first had RA. An avid golfer, he felt the first pangs of pain in his shoulder, which he brushed off as a sports-related injury. Then the pain would appear in the other shoulder, only to disappear in both shoulders a few weeks later.

In 2002, he started noticing what he calls transitory inflammation around his body, especially in his arms and wrists. The inflammation was painful, but it would typically go away, then return in his shoulders again.

While working with a personal trainer that summer, Bruce noticed he couldn't lift his hand above his shoulder. This time, the pain persisted and surfaced in the other shoulder. He went to a rheumatologist, who diagnosed him as having RA and gave him Plaquenil. The pain intensified. "I couldn't reach back far enough to put my coat on," he says. "I had to go downstairs and get the doorman to help. You're like a two-year-old when you can't even put your own coat on."

One day, his hip got so inflamed that he couldn't get to work and had to use a cane and a car service. Another time, while on vacation in Turkey, he was wracked with so much pain that he couldn't get out of bed. "I have a fairly high threshold for pain," he says. "But I can remember sitting in a chair, and my wrist hurt so bad that I was crying."

After trying prednisone and methotrexate, Bruce finally found relief about a year ago with Enbrel. "Within two weeks, the Enbrel started working," he says. "Basically, I now have no arthritis symptoms."

Once a week, the former Army medic gives himself an injection using a needle that's less than a half-inch long. "I've had allergy injections for fifty years, so these don't hurt," he says. He keeps his medication in the refrigerator and stores it in an insulated bag if he's on the road.

The relief has allowed Bruce to continue doing all the activities he loves—downhill skiing, golfing, cross-country skiing, biking, and running. "I'm lucky and I know it," Bruce says. "I assume at some point the RA could come back. But as long as I can do what I want to do, I'm fine."

CHAPTER NINE ❧

Surgical Options

You've tried several medications, but nothing has helped to control your pain and inflammation. Frustration sets in, and you may begin to wonder about surgery. Can it help alleviate your pain and restore the function to your joints?

Surgery to treat RA may provide temporary relief from the pain and swelling, and prevent further damage to the joints. It may also be done as a corrective measure to improve the function of joints already damaged by the disease. In addition, surgery can repair ruptured ligaments or tendons, remove inflamed synovial tissue, and restore or retain function of a joint that's losing mobility.

Making the decision to have surgery is often not an easy task. It helps to understand your options, the benefits and risks of having or not having surgery, and the recovery that will be involved as you heal.

DO I NEED SURGERY?
Perhaps you've been unable to sleep at night because of persistent pain. Maybe you've tried numerous medications and had no relief. Or perhaps the medication you're taking has stopped working for

you. Maybe you're finding that your ability to get around has become severely restricted to the point where getting out of a chair or climbing stairs has become difficult.

If you've been experiencing any of these difficulties, you may be wondering if you're a candidate for surgery. The first step is a conversation with your doctor, probably your rheumatologist. Your physician can help you determine whether surgery can help your situation. People with certain medical conditions, such as those with cardiac disease, renal disease, or lung disease, for instance, may be at increased risk for complications from surgery.

If you think you might benefit from surgery, or your doctor has raised the possibility, you should gather some information before making a decision. According to the Arthritis Foundation, there are several questions you should ask when talking to your doctor about surgery. They include:

- What are my other options besides surgery?
- Can you explain the operation in detail?
- How long will the surgery take?
- What are the risks involved in the procedure? How likely am I to experience them?
- What options are available to avoid blood transfusions?
- What type of anesthesia is involved? What are the risks?
- Will more surgery be needed?
- Who will do my surgery?
- What are your qualifications for performing the surgery? What is your experience? Are you board-certified?
- Can you give me the name of someone else who has undergone this surgery and is willing to talk to me about it?
- Is exercise recommended after the surgery?
- Do I need to stop taking any of my medications before surgery?

- What happens if I delay surgery? What are the risks of not having the surgery?
- How long will I remain in the hospital?
- How much pain will I experience after surgery? Will I receive medication for the pain? How long will the pain last?
- When do I start physical therapy? Will I need home or outpatient therapy?
- Do you have written materials or videos about postoperative care?
- Will I need to arrange assistance for at-home care?
- Will I need special equipment at home?
- What medications will I need at home? How long will I need to take them?
- What limits will I have on my daily activities such as driving, climbing stairs, and having sex?
- How often will I have follow-up visits with you?

Also be sure to check with your health insurance provider to find out whether your in-hospital rehabilitation is covered. Also, will your health insurance cover any home health care? Does it cover physical therapy? Occupational therapy?

WHO WILL PERFORM THE SURGERY?

Different specialties allow surgeons—like other medical professionals—to specialize in different types of surgery. Orthopedic surgeons, for instance, do surgery on bones and joints. Some may perform surgery only on large joints like the shoulders, knees, elbows, and hips, but others may also have expertise in surgeries of small joints like those of the hands and feet. Orthopedic surgeons may also specialize in joint reconstruction or arthroscopic surgery.

If you need surgery on your hand, you may need a hand surgeon. Hand surgeons are highly specialized experts, with training in orthopedic surgery or plastic surgery. Similarly, if you need surgery on your feet, you may need a foot and ankle orthopedic surgeon, who is trained to treat foot ailments and also perform foot surgery.

TYPES OF SURGERY

Different types of damage require different kinds of surgery. Here are the surgical procedures most often used to correct the damaging effects of RA.

Arthrodesis

When joints become painful and unstable, your physician may recommend a joint fusion, also called arthrodesis. Most of these procedures are done on joints in the ankles, wrists, fingers, and thumbs. The two bones that form the joint are joined together, so that the joint becomes less flexible. Because motion becomes permanently restricted, this procedure is rarely done on the shoulder or hips. Though movement is inhibited, the procedure does help relieve pain and improve stability.

Arthroscopy

Using a tool called an arthroscope, which is a thin tube with a light at the end, an orthopedist can look directly into the joint through a small incision in the skin. The arthroscope is attached to a closed-circuit television and lets the physician assess the extent of the damage to the cartilage, synovial lining, and ligaments. This procedure is most commonly performed on knees and shoulders. It can also be used to repair ligaments and tendons. Most often, it's used to perform a synovectomy.

Synovectomy

When the joint lining, or synovium, becomes inflamed, it may cause damage to the cartilage and other tissues in the joints. To prevent that, your doctor may recommend a synovectomy. Synovectomies are most often performed on the knees, elbows, and wrists. The procedure reduces pain and swelling, and can slow the destruction of the joints. Unfortunately, however, complete removal of the synovium is not possible, and the synovium often grows back several years later, causing the pain and problems to recur.

Synovectomy may be performed through an arthroscope, which allows the surgeon to avoid cutting and opening the joint capsule. As a result, recovery from an arthroscopic synovectomy is often fairly quick. An open surgical synovectomy, on the other hand, results in a longer recovery period but gives the surgeon a better view and greater access to the whole joint, making it easier for him to remove more of the synovial tissue.

Most patients will be given an antibiotic during the procedure to prevent infection. After a synovectomy, you may need to wear a sling or a splint, depending on the joint that was operated on. You will also undergo physical therapy and take pain management medications.

Tenosynovectomy

RA can damage tendon sheaths, causing them to swell and restricting the movement of the joint. The removal of the inflamed tendons is called a tenosynovectomy. In patients with RA, this procedure is most commonly done on the wrists, the hands, or the feet.

Tendon Transfer and Reconstruction

In some patients, RA may cause a tendon to rupture, making them unable to extend or straighten out their fingers. If that occurs, your doctor may suggest a tendon transfer. Many tendons have an associated tendon that can perform the same function, which makes it possible to borrow a tendon and transfer it to another tendon.

When the tendon with the functioning muscle is attached to the end of the tendon that's ruptured, the patient's finger function can be restored. Tendons in the tops of the hands that travel to the fingers are most vulnerable to rupture.

After the surgery, physical therapy is often prescribed and is often best done by an experienced hand therapist. Often, special splints are required to control the hand position while the hand heals.

Osteotomy

If deformity occurs in the bones, a surgeon may be enlisted to perform an osteotomy. This procedure involves cutting and repositioning the bone to improve joint alignment and compensate for the deformity. Osteotomy is usually done in people whose joints have fallen out of alignment and who have mild osteoarthritis. It is also used in people who are too young for total hip replacement. But as joint replacement procedures have been improved, osteotomies have become less common.

In some cases, a section of the bone is removed from the end nearest the joint, a procedure that is called bone resection. This simple procedure is usually done in the shoulders, elbows, wrists, and feet to improve the range of motion and to relieve pain.

Arthroplasty

In some patients, a joint may become severely damaged, raising the prospect of arthroplasty, also called joint replacement. This procedure may involve rebuilding the joint, which is achieved by resurfacing or relining the ends of the bones where the cartilage has eroded and the bone has been destroyed. In some cases, it may involve realigning the joint. Or, it may mean replacing the entire damaged joint with an artificial one.

Artificial joints were first introduced about forty years ago and have undergone major improvements since. Today's artificial joints are usually made of a mix of metal—usually stainless steel or alloys—and plastic. Some of the new implants used for hip replacement are made of a special ceramic material or oxidized zirconium, which has a smooth surface that reduces the wear that often requires revision surgery. These sturdier implants may last up to twenty-five years; older replacements may last fifteen years.

Total joint replacement is typically done in the knees, hips, and shoulders and met with success. In the hands, elbows, wrists, and ankles, the outcome has been less predictable, so the procedure is done less frequently in these joints.

In the hips and knees, the artificial joint may be attached in one of two ways:

- **Cemented joint replacement.** In this version, the surgeon drills a hole in the existing bone and attaches the artificial joint by inserting the stem into the hole. Recovery from this type of procedure is generally quicker and less painful, but over time, the cement may crack and loosen, especially if you're active. This procedure might be better for older, less active patients, though improvements in the cement have made it viable for younger people, too.
- **Cementless joint replacement.** Patients whose artificial joints are attached without cement are fitted with components that fit inside the bone. These components are made of a porous material, which allows the natural bone to grow into it. The replacement stem is inserted into a hole in the bone, and it's up to the patient's bone to grow and provide newfound stability. Recovery may take longer since the bone needs to grow. But the patient usually experiences more strength and durability in the artificial joint and is less likely to need surgery later.

Not everyone can get a cementless joint replacement, however. People who have osteoporosis, a condition marked by porous bones, for instance, are not good candidates since the bones will need to grow into the prosthesis. And if RA has already weakened your bones, cementless joint replacement may not be viable.

What Kind of Arthroplasty Will I Get?

The type of joint replacement you get will depend in part on where you need the surgery. Cemented replacements, for instance, may work better on knees. If you need a hip replacement in the upper part of your leg, the cementless version may be better. In patients who get hip replacements, surgeons sometimes do a combination of the two variations. Other factors that can determine the type of arthroplasty you'll get include your age, weight, and the shape of your bones.

After having joint replacement, you will need several weeks to recover, no matter which procedure you get. Patients usually experience improvement by six weeks, but the recovery process continues for several months. They also experience less pain in the affected joint and improvement in their ability to function.

Talk to your doctor at length about your job, lifestyle, and exercise habits before you have joint replacement done. Find out how long you'll need to abstain from your normal activities. The rehabilitation process varies for everyone. For instance, if your job is physically demanding, you may need to stay out of work for a longer period of time than if you have a desk job. And if you are younger and in good shape before the surgery, you may recover more quickly than an older patient who is sedentary.

Recently, some patients have been benefiting from the use of minimally invasive surgical techniques during joint replacement surgery. These techniques involve less cutting, less trauma, less blood loss, and a more rapid recovery.

Considerations Before Arthroplasty

Getting joint replacement surgery is a major decision, and it's not for everyone. The recovery period is lengthy and requires a strong commitment to physical therapy. On top of that, surgery is expensive.

On the other hand, surgery can do wonders to alleviate your pain and restore the movement in the affected joint. It can also help improve the quality of your life.

Clearly, there are benefits to getting arthroplasty. But some people do not make good candidates for arthroplasty. Before going forward with surgery, be sure to consider the following:

- **Your health.** Certain health conditions might make surgery more difficult for you. For instance, if you have cardiovascular disease or lung problems, surgery could be too taxing. If you take immunosuppressant drugs, you may be at greater risk for infection during surgery.

    Some surgeries may pose a greater risk to your health. For instance, hip and knee replacement surgeries are more likely to cause blood clots. Your surgeon will typically prescribe an anti-clotting medication to prevent this from happening.
- **Your weight.** Being overweight is another burden that might interfere with your having surgery. Weighing too much can also slow the recovery process and increase the risk of complications. RA patients are vulnerable to weight gain because the arthritis may limit their mobility and function, and some medications like steroids might cause them to gain weight.
- **Your age.** By itself, age does not make someone ineligible for surgery, but elderly patients may be more likely to have other conditions that might put them at greater risk for surgical complications. Conversely, sometimes an artificial

joint may not last as long in a young, active patient as it would in an older, sedentary patient. The artificial joint is more likely to wear out more quickly in a younger patient who puts extra stress on it.

- **The recovery process.** Getting the surgery is only part of the equation in terms of gaining any benefits from the procedure. As the patient, you must be strongly committed to bringing about your recovery. That means diligently doing the postsurgical exercises that are prescribed to you, making follow-up appointments with health-care professionals, and taking the necessary medications. If you're not committed, surgery may not be for you. In that case, the surgery is not likely to be a success.

- **The costs.** No doubt, arthroplasty is an expensive procedure. The total cost will vary depending on various factors including the surgeon, the anesthesiologist, hospital, medication, types of implants, and any special tests or treatments. Before having surgery done, it's a good idea to find out what your health insurance plan covers.

YOUR PRESURGERY TO-DO LIST

At your doctor's advice, you've decided to go ahead and get surgery. In order to ensure that the surgery is a success, there are things you should do beforehand. Consider this your to-do list:

- Discuss the medications you are taking with your rheumatologist. Your rheumatologist may want to change your medication regimen in the weeks leading up to surgery.
- Tell your surgeon about every medication you're taking, especially nonsteroidal anti-inflammatories, corticosteroids, DMARDs, and biologics. Even over-the-counter NSAIDS pose a risk for bleeding, so be sure to mention the occasional

ibuprofen or aspirin. Your surgeon should also know about any immunosuppression drugs you're taking, such as methotrexate, cyclosporine, etanercept, and anakinra.

- Discuss options for potential blood replacement. If you need a blood transfusion during surgery and want to receive your own blood, arrange to have your blood set aside beforehand, which is known as an autologous transfusion.
- Be honest about your health. If you develop an infection around the time of your surgery, you need to tell your surgeon beforehand. An infection in any part of the body can travel by way of the bloodstream to the artificial joint and cause an infection there. You also need to tell your physician about severe dental cavities. Problems in the teeth or gums can increase your risk for infection, so it's best to have dental matters treated before getting surgery.
- Get in the habit of eating well-balanced meals before surgery. Take a daily multivitamin with iron, too. Eating well will help you recover.
- Stop or reduce smoking. Ideally, you should quit altogether.
- Prepare your home for your post-surgery recovery. Pin down loose carpets, tape down electrical cords, and remove stray objects that could interfere with your getting around safely. Place things you use frequently within easy reach. If necessary, install assistive devices around the house, such as handrails in the tub or shower. Make sure to have a stable chair with firm cushioning and armrests in the room or rooms where you'll spend most days.
- Arrange for help. Ask relatives, friends, and neighbors to help with simple tasks, like cooking, shopping, and laundry, if possible. To make food preparation easier, make meals beforehand and keep them in the freezer.

In the week or so before surgery, you'll be given a full physical examination to determine your overall health. You'll also be given routine tests such as X-rays and blood tests. If you're taking aspirin or another blood-thinning medication, you'll be asked to stop a week before the surgery.

The better prepared you are beforehand, the more energy you'll have for participating in your recovery. And that will certainly enhance your odds for a successful surgery.

AFTER SURGERY

The recovery period after surgery varies depending on the surgery you had and the joint that was operated on. But in general, all patients are prescribed rest, physical therapy, and limited activity.

As soon as you're able, you'll be required to participate in physical therapy. The exercises you do will be challenging, possibly even painful, as you begin to work muscles that haven't been working as hard or have been working improperly because of a bad joint. The good news is that the difficulty of these exercises will eventually ease up as you continue to do them and your muscles get stronger. Eventually, you may even get bored by these exercises and feel tempted to slack off. Don't! The key to a successful recovery is following the instructions of your physical therapist. You'll be rewarded with greater mobility, less pain, and improved functioning.

PROFILE

DONNA

When Donna first developed rheumatoid arthritis at the age of twenty-seven, her doctors were convinced she simply had a case of tendonitis or carpal tunnel syndrome. After all, she was working at a job that involved a lot of typing, and the pain was in her wrists and arms. "My whole arm would throb, and I didn't know what was going on," she says. "But then it went away."

Not long after that, she developed a pain in her shoulder, which doctors said was bursitis, inflammation of the fluid-filled sacs, or bursae, near the shoulder joint. The pain lasted a month or two, then, again, subsided.

The next symptom emerged in her feet. Every morning when she awoke, her feet were swollen. As the day wore on, the swelling went away, and again, Donna was relieved.

When the aches in her wrists returned, Donna began doing her own research. She stumbled on information about RA and realized that a lot of the symptoms she was reading about applied to her. A friend gave her the name of a rheumatologist, who diagnosed her with RA.

At first, Donna took the news in stride and figured she'd simply push past the disease. "I was doing theater at night and working at a job during the day," says Donna, now fifty-five. "My doctor told me that the disease was going to progress and that I needed to rest. But I didn't really believe him. When you're twenty-seven, you think nothing can hurt you."

Her rheumatologist's prediction proved to be right. While working for a woman she describes as a terrible boss, Donna came under enormous stress. The pain from RA worsened. Her legs and feet became extremely swollen, and Donna couldn't even find shoes that fit. The worst pain was in her knees, which caused Donna to limp. After a year, she finally quit the job and began experimenting with various DMARDs, such as gold, methotrexate, Plaquenil, and minocycline.

The drugs did help, but Donna was still in constant pain. While she worked in media relations and gave tours of the company facility at a new job, Donna had to use a cane. She also couldn't straighten her right arm because her elbow was crooked. In the late 1980s, she had a synovectomy to remove the synovium in her right elbow. Fortunately, it restored the mobility in her arm.

But the pain in her knees persisted. In 1993, she finally had surgery to replace her right knee. "It had gotten very painful to walk," she says. "I couldn't even get up and down from a chair. When I saw the X-rays, I could see that it was bone on bone, and that the cartilage had completely eroded."

Recovery was long and difficult. It took six weeks before Donna could return to work because she couldn't drive. Donna later learned that the replacement knee was slightly crooked, and that the surgery had been performed by a med school resident, not the highly recommended surgeon she'd enlisted. "I do still have pain in my right knee sometimes," she says.

The first knee surgery was followed three years later with shoulder surgery on her left side. Donna had been experiencing pain near her neck. The X-ray showed that half her shoulder joint had completely eroded away. The surgeon did what he could to repair the shoulder, but her range of motion was still limited. Even now, years after the surgery and subsequent recovery, Donna still has trouble raising her left arm as high as her right.

That same year, Donna had surgery on her left knee, this time with another surgeon who assured her that he would be doing the surgery. Fortunately, the recovery was much faster than it had been after the first knee surgery, and Donna was walking with a cane in a week and a half.

These days, Donna's knees still impose some restrictions. At church, she does not kneel with the rest of the congregation. Rather than kneel in the dirt when she gardens, she sits on a tiny bench. And as an actress in local theater troupes, she cannot take on roles that involve excessive kneeling or frequent trips up and down stairs.

Her indomitable spirit and energy, she says, is what has helped her survive the surgeries and the challenges of RA. "My doctor says that what's kept me going all these years in spite of the severity of my RA is that I've always looked forward to things," she notes. "I'm always involved and looking for things to do."

In addition to acting, Donna is active in publicity and fundraising for the American Autoimmune Related Diseases Association. She also sings in the church choir and sits on the church council.

A couple of years ago, she also started going to a gym, where she walks on a treadmill and does strength training. Besides helping to tame her pain, the effort helped her shed twenty pounds. "There are times when I know I can't do a lot," she says. "But you have to know when you can push past the pain and when you can't."

Donna also credits her spirituality and positive attitude with helping her survive RA. "I go to church a lot, and I surround myself with a lot of other spiritual people," she says. "And I've learned not to hold grudges, to just let it out and get over it. I also try to laugh as much as I can."

CHAPTER TEN ✤

Alternative Treatments for RA

These days, more Americans than ever are looking at alternative medicines as an option for treating their ailments—everything from back pain to depression. According to a 2004 report by the National Center for Complementary and Alternative Medicine (NCCAM) and the National Center for Health Statistics, 36 percent of adults age eighteen and older use some form of complementary medicine. If you count prayer and megavitamin therapy, that number rises to 62 percent. Spending on these alternative therapies is estimated at almost fifty billion dollars.

Why the rising popularity? According to the NCCAM study, many people turn to alternative therapies as a way to complement their conventional treatments or because conventional therapies didn't work. Those studied also cited an interest in alternative remedies and an effort to avoid the high cost of conventional treatments.

When you are suffering from the pains of RA and waiting for relief from conventional medicine, you, too, may be tempted to give alternative remedies a try. You may consider massage as a way to knead away your pain. You may consider taking glucosamine and chondroitin to ease the aches in your joints. You may turn to valerian as a way to get the sleep that eludes you when you're experiencing pain in bed at night.

Before you delve into the world of alternative remedies, make sure to talk to your physician and do your research. RA is not a disease that can be treated by alternative remedies, though some therapies might provide some additional relief. Like all aspects of this condition, the key is knowing as much as possible.

SAFETY CONSIDERATIONS

You see an ad on the Internet for a supplement that promises to alleviate joint aches. Your cousin tells you of his success using supplements to improve his sleep. A colleague tells you of an acupuncturist who cured him of his anxieties. Should you pursue these leads in treating your RA?

Truth is, research on many alternative therapies is rare—though that may be changing—so there is often little scientific proof to back up claims made about alternative products and therapies. Each treatment needs to be considered on its own merits and how it might impact your health. But you should know some general guidelines:

- Natural does not automatically mean safe. Many supplements are touted as being "natural," implying that they are somehow superior to treatments produced in a lab. But natural is not the same as safe. For instance, wild mushrooms and berries are natural, but many of them are poisonous.
- Everyone responds differently to different treatments. The state of your health, how the treatment is used, and your belief in the treatment can all impact how well a remedy works for you. Just because your brother benefited from the use of acupuncture for his backaches doesn't mean massage will cure you of the aches in your shoulders.

• The safety of over-the-counter supplements is primarily in the hands of the manufacturer. Supplements are classified as food, not as drugs. The U.S. Food and Drug Administration (FDA) regulates dietary supplements under the Dietary Supplement Health and Education Act of 1994 (DSHEA), which says the dietary supplement manufacturer is responsible for ensuring that a supplement is safe before it is marketed. The safety depends on several factors, including the ingredients, where they come from, and the quality of the manufacturing process. Manufacturers must also make sure that information on the product label is truthful and not misleading.

   That means most manufacturers do not need to register with the FDA nor get FDA approval before producing or selling dietary supplements. The FDA is responsible, however, for taking action against any unsafe dietary supplement product after it reaches the market. So if a product is deemed unsafe, the FDA can prohibit its sale.

• Claims that a supplement can diagnose, treat, cure, or prevent disease are invalid unless scientific proof is provided. Any manufacturer that tries to sell a product with these kinds of promises and has no scientific evidence to back them up is violating government regulations. Without scientific proof behind these claims, the product is considered an unapproved drug and is therefore being sold illegally.

• Alternative therapies that are administered by a practitioner depend in large part on the training, skill, and experience of the practitioner. However, in spite of careful and skilled practice, all treatments can have risks. The key is to minimize yours by choosing a practitioner carefully. Ask your health-care team for recommendations, contact a local professional organization, or talk to others who have gotten these services.

DOING THE RESEARCH

It's a good idea to do your own research so you can understand a treatment's risks and potential benefits. Here are some ways to find that information:

Talk to Your Health-Care Practitioners

Tell your health-care team about the therapy you are considering and ask about its safety, effectiveness, and interactions with medications you're taking. Even if your doctor can't give you specifics about the therapy, he might be able to refer you to someone who can. You can also ask your doctor to interpret some of the information you do find.

Surf the Web for Information

The Internet may be the source of some outlandish health claims, but it's also a wonderful resource for getting information about specific treatments, alternative and otherwise. Some good places to check include:

- *The NCCAM Web site at nccam.nih.gov.* Search for information about specific therapies. Check out whether there are new or ongoing studies into the treatment. If you don't have Internet access, call the NCCAM clearinghouse at 888-644-6226.
- *The FDA at www.fda.gov.* Check here to see if there is any information available about the product or practice. If you're looking into dietary supplements, check out the FDA's Center for Food Safety and Applied Nutrition Web site at www.cfsan.fda.gov. Or visit the FDA's Web page on recalls and safety alerts at www.fda.gov/opacom/7alerts.html.
- *The Federal Trade Commission (FTC) at www.ftc.gov.* Look to see if there are any fraudulent claims or consumer alerts

regarding the therapy. Visit the Diet, Health, and Fitness Consumer Information Web site at www.ftc.gov/bcp/menu-health.htm.

- *CAM on PubMed at www.nlm.nih.gov/nccam/camonpubmed.html.* Developed by NCCAM and the National Library of Medicine, this Web site gives citations or abstracts (brief summaries) of the results of scientific studies on alternative therapies. In some cases, it provides links to publishers' Web sites where you may be able to view or obtain the full articles. The articles cited in CAM on PubMed have been reviewed by other scientists in the same field, something known as peer review. These scientists have read the article, examined the data and conclusions, and judged them to be accurate and important.

- *The International Bibliographic Information on Dietary Supplements database at http://ods.od.nih.gov/Health_Information/IBIDS.aspx.* This Web site is useful for searching the scientific literature on dietary supplements.

When using a Web site, check to see that the operator of the site is the government, a university, or a reputable medical or health-related association. Be wary if it's sponsored by a company that manufactures the supplement or has something to gain by peddling it. Also, be sure the information you're reading is current, up-to-date, and based on scientific evidence. The material should present clear references to back it up, not opinions.

MINIMIZE YOUR RISKS

Assume you do decide to try an alternative treatment to complement your conventional medication regimen. Maybe the idea of acupuncture is appealing to you, or the thought of a massage is promising. Like any treatment, every alternative remedy may pose some risk. That doesn't mean you shouldn't use them; it just means you need to always be aware of how you can minimize the risks.

If you do decide to try alternative therapies, alert everyone involved on your health-care team that you are considering or are using the therapy. This is critical to your safety. For instance, certain herbal or botanical products and dietary supplements may interact with medications. They may also have negative, even dangerous, effects on their own. For instance, ginkgo, which is used to improve circulation, may be dangerous if you're taking a blood-thinning medication like aspirin. And kava, an herb that has been used for insomnia, stress, and anxiety, has been linked to liver damage.

TREATMENTS YOU MAY CONSIDER

Now that you've been properly warned about the risks involved in getting alternative therapies, you may want to know about specific remedies that have helped people with RA. Most of these are not backed by scientific studies, though some alternative remedies may provide actual relief for people with RA. Just remember, if you do decide to try a nonconventional treatment, be sure to tell your health-care providers. It certainly cannot replace your need for conventional medications and treatments.

Massage

The manual manipulation of soft body tissues is known as massage. Rubbing, kneading, rolling, and pressing the tissue increases blood flow and warmth.

Massage is generally not an option for someone in the throes of a severe flare-up of RA. You may simply be too sore or swollen to have massage. But if your condition is mild to moderate, ask your physician about getting a massage.

When you do get a massage, be sure to tell the massage therapist that you have RA and to identify the joints that are most affected.

You may want to specify a Swedish massage, which is gentler than other forms of massage and focuses on gently stroking and kneading the skin to enhance circulation and muscle relaxation. Other massage techniques like deep tissue massage and myofascial are more rigorous and may be too painful for someone with RA. But no matter what technique you receive, be sure to alert the therapist to any pain you feel.

Acupuncture and Acupressure

The use of acupuncture dates back thousands of years in ancient China. Tiny needles are inserted into the skin along meridian lines on the body, which correspond to various organs. The procedure works by opening up the pathways of qi, or life energy, and restoring health.

In the United States, acupuncture has undergone a revival of sorts and is now a popular method for alleviating all kinds of pain. The procedure may be used to relieve migraines, to enhance fertility, and to alleviate depression. In reality, though, acupuncture does little for RA, except to provide some temporary relief from the pain. However, it may induce relaxation and help promote sleep, which can, in turn, lessen the pain in RA. And animal studies show that acupuncture increases levels of cortisol, which is a natural anti-inflammatory agent in the body.

For people who do not like needles, acupressure offers an alternative. The practice involves the same principles as acupuncture, namely restoring harmonious flow of qi throughout the body in order to improve health. But instead of needles, the procedure involves the use of the practitioner's hands.

If you do decide to try acupuncture or acupressure, find a licensed therapist. Tell your doctor of your plans to make sure you're healthy enough. Be honest with the acupuncturist about your health; he should be told of your RA as well as any other conditions and any medications you take. If your acupuncturist recommends herbal supplements, talk to your doctor first before taking them. They could cause dangerous interactions. Also, keep track of your progress. Acupuncture may require four to six sessions before it takes effect.

Tai Chi

Patients with RA who want to improve their range of motion may find some benefits from doing tai chi, a practice that combines slow, gentle flowing movements with concentration and deep breathing. Some call it meditation in motion. Tai chi emerged sometime in the 1300s to 1600s in China. Participants shift their weight through a series of controlled movements that flow from one move to the next. Like acupuncture, tai chi is intended to balance the flow of qi.

Studies suggest that tai chi may have beneficial effects on hypertension, multiple sclerosis, and falls in the elderly. A study published in 2004 found that tai chi improved range of motion of the lower extremities among RA patients, especially in the ankle. But the study did not evaluate improvements in the pain or in quality of life.

If you are interested in trying tai chi, find a qualified teacher who can work with patients who have arthritis. If necessary, modify the movements to minimize your pain. Never overexert yourself, and stop if you experience pain.

Homeopathy

Homeopathy is a healing system based on the notion that small amounts of the disease-causing substance can actually trigger a curative response, much in the same way that vaccinations use mild amounts of a disease in order to trigger an immune system response. It was developed in the eighteenth century by a German physician who went on to create thousands of remedies derived from herbs, minerals, and animal products.

Today, homeopathy is highly individualized. A homeopathic doctor takes a detailed history of your lifestyle, symptoms, and preferences, and then creates a remedy for you using a vast data bank of natural remedies. Sometimes, a single remedy is used. Other times, it is a combination of remedies. Often, for mild conditions such as a cold, consumers can self-treat and purchase homeopathic remedies in health food stores, pharmacies, or grocery stores.

As of now, there is no scientific evidence that homeopathy can help relieve the symptoms of RA. Some doctors may be willing to use homeopathy to complement conventional treatments, but never to replace them. If you want to consider homeopathy, talk to your doctor first. And don't abandon the use of conventional medications for homeopathy.

Chiropractics

Manipulating the spine as a way to improve your health is at the root of chiropractic care, one of the oldest healing practices still in existence. Spinal manipulation was described by Hippocrates in ancient Greece. Modern chiropractic care was developed in 1895 by Daniel David Palmer in Davenport, Iowa. Palmer believed that the body had a natural healing ability that was controlled by the nervous system. He also believed that misalignments of the spine, also called subluxations, interrupted or interfered with this "nerve flow." If an organ doesn't get its normal supply of impulses from the nerves, he believed, it can become diseased. To correct that, he developed a procedure to adjust the bones of the spinal column.

These days, people visit chiropractors for numerous ailments, including colds, allergies, and aches and pains. But if you have RA, you should be very cautious about trying chiropractics. Manipulation of the spine or any other joint in a patient who has RA can be harmful and damaging.

Supplements

It would be appealing to think that taking an all-natural remedy could halt a disease and its symptoms, without any impact from side effects. And indeed, Americans do find the use of supplements appealing. According to the *Nutrition Business Journal,* sales of herbal supplements totaled $4.2 billion in 2003.

But when it comes to RA, there is no scientific proof that supplements help, though some products do offer promise. Common ones you may have heard about include:

Fish Oil

Studies suggest that fish oil may help reduce the pain and swelling in RA. Experts believe that the omega-3 fatty acids—specifically eicosapentaenoic (EPA) and docosahexaenoic (DHA) acids—found in fish oil help reduce inflammation. Studies have shown that in patients with mild, stable RA, fish oil supplements did in fact lower their inflammation and allow them to reduce their dosage of NSAIDs. However, fish oil does not appear to have any advantages over NSAIDs, and it does not slow the progression of the disease the way DMARDs and biologics can.

The best way to get your omega-3 fatty acids is to eat more fish, as discussed in chapter five. Good options include sardines, salmon, anchovy, mackerel, herring, and lake trout. Omega-3 fatty acids are also present in olive and flaxseed oils. Be careful about taking fish oil supplements since fish oil does have a blood-thinning effect.

Gamma Linolenic Acid (GLA)

Also known as omega-6 fatty acid, GLA is another fatty acid that might have benefits for RA patients. Like omega-3 fatty acids, it appears to reduce inflammation. GLA does not occur in large quantities in food, so you'll need to get it from supplements, such as evening primrose oil, black currant oil, and borage oil. Be sure to tell your doctor if you take these supplements because GLA may interact with blood-thinning medications.

Glucosamine Sulfate and Chondroitin
Both of these substances are part of natural human cartilage. As supplements, glucosamine is derived from shellfish, and chondroitin from pigs. People who have osteoarthritis have reaped the benefits of these two supplements, which help alleviate the pain and stiffness caused by wear and tear on the cartilage. But glucosamine and chondroitin generally don't help people with RA, whose pain and stiffness is brought on by inflammation.

Other Supplements
Lesser-known supplements may also have some anti-inflammatory effects on the body, and may even reduce pain and swelling. These include the following:

- **Boswellia** is an herb used in the traditional Ayurvedic medicine of India. It is considered an anti-inflammatory.
- **Bovine cartilage** is a supplement made from the ground cartilage of cow trachea or windpipes. It may help resynthesize human cartilage and may have anti-inflammatory effects.
- **Bromelain** is an enzyme in pineapple juice that breaks down protein, which may relieve pain and inflammation.
- **Cat's claw** is the dried root bark of a woody vine from the Amazon rain forests of Peru that may have anti-inflammatory effects.
- **Cetyl-myristoleate** is a waxy fatlike substance derived from mice that may help lubricate joints. It's also believed to regulate the immune system and control inflammation.
- **Collagen hydrolysate** is a protein in cartilage that is derived from pigs, cows, ox, chicken, or sheep. It may relieve

the pain, inflammation, swelling, and stiffness of RA and other diseases.

- **Devil's claw** is derived from the root of an African plant and is used in Europe as an anti-inflammatory for people with RA.
- **Ginger** is a spice that comes from the dried or fresh root of the ginger plant, commonly used in cooking. Its ingredients may produce an analgesic effect and reduce inflammation.
- **Ginseng** is derived from the root of the ginseng plant found in North America and Asia. The herb is believed to help alleviate stress and fatigue, and enhance immune function, stamina, and cognitive function.
- **Gotu-kola,** also called Indian pennywort, is a plant that grows in parts of Asia and South Africa. It is believed to reduce fatigue and pain, improve circulation, and ease the symptoms of RA.
- **Grapeseed** comes from the seeds of grapes from a woody vine native to Asia Minor. It may reduce inflammation, improve circulation, and combat fatigue.
- **Green tea** comes from the leaves of the tea plant in southeast Asia. The tea contains polyphenols, which are antioxidants that combat inflammation.
- **Thunder God vine** comes from the leaf and root of a vinelike plant in Asia. A small study published in 2002 found that an extract of the root reduced pain and inflammation in people whose RA had resisted other forms of treatment.
- **Turmeric** is powder ground from the turmeric plant, which also produces curry powder. It is believed to reduce inflammation and stiffness in RA. Curcumin, an extract of turmeric, is also used as a supplement.
- **Valerian** comes from the root of the plant by the same name. The remedy is intended to promote sleep and ease muscle aches and pain.

A Warning about Supplements

It's easy to be lulled into a false sense of security by something that's labeled "natural." But herbs and supplements can have dangerous interactions with prescription and over-the-counter remedies. Bromelain, for instance, may increase the effects of blood-thinning drugs. Echinacea, an herb often associated with treating colds, can counteract immune-suppressant medications such as glucocorticoids. GLA may enhance the effects of aspirin and other blood-thinning medications.

That's why it's so important to tell your doctor about any supplement you're considering. Just because something is natural doesn't necessarily mean it's good for you. Even zinc, an essential mineral, can interfere with glucocorticoids and immune-suppressing drugs. So learn the side effects of the supplements before you embark on any experiments with them.

BEWARE OF QUACKERY

The quest for relief is urgent when you're battling the ravages of RA at its worst, especially if you've tried several treatments and experienced no relief. Promises of quick, easy cures sound appealing when all you want is to extinguish the pain and become healthy again.

Certain phrases may sound particularly appealing when you're in such a desperate position. The FDA advises that some words and phrases may actually disguise a lack of science such as "innovation," "quick cure," "miracle cure," "exclusive product," "new discovery," or "magical discovery."

Be on the lookout for these phrases and for claims of a "secret formula." If ever a therapy was discovered that could cure RA, surely it would be widely reported, prescribed, and recommended. Also, be suspicious of conspiracy claims that a particular treatment has been suppressed by the government or the medical community.

These are usually meant to divert you to another treatment. Finally, be wary of claims that a treatment can cure a wide range of unrelated conditions, such as a supplement that can treat cancer, diabetes, and AIDS. There is simply no product that can treat every disease and condition.

It's dangerous to experiment with untested remedies, which at best may do nothing and at worst may cause even more damage. In addition, it is costly and time-consuming, and can give you false hopes for a quick cure.

Whether you decide to use alternative remedies is ultimately up to you. But remember, it's important to stay on the course that your rheumatologist prescribes and to continue taking the recommended medications.

PROFILE

PAT

By any account, Pat was a high-energy woman, a single mom who had worked in the fashion industry and the corporate world, held three or four jobs at a time, and then struck out on her own to start an international marketing consulting company. She slept no more than three or four hours a night and traveled around the world for her work. She was on what she calls a "treadmill running full speed" all her life.

Her world began to change at the age of forty-eight, when she started experiencing symptoms of rheumatoid arthritis. One day she awoke with her face swollen. Then she started to experience swelling in her hands, knees, or hips. A rash on her face refused to go away. Pat was puzzled and concerned.

"I didn't know what was happening to me at first," she says. "I was not able to eat or sleep. I had great difficulty bending, and getting up when I sat for more than fifteen minutes. I had severe headaches that were debilitating, and I had gained fifteen pounds."

Blood tests revealed nothing, so Pat began a two-year quest for a diagnosis and a doctor. In the interim, she saw more than fifteen physicians. Some doctors she tried to see told her up front that they could not help her. "I went to rheumatologists, oncologists, neurologists, immunologists, endocrinologists, internists, dermatologists, and regular medical doctors," she says. "They all prescribed the same therapy—steroids."

By the time she found her doctor, Richard Ash, an internist in Manhattan—Pat wants her doctors to get full credit—she was in terrible condition. She could no longer drive because she couldn't grip the steering wheel. She couldn't wear shoes with backs on them because she could no longer bend her feet. She slept on a medical air mattress to help her get out of bed in the morning. She couldn't get in or out of a shower or tub without assistance.

Typing on a computer was impossible because it hurt to peck the keys. Getting out of a chair was undoable without help. Cooking, a long-time passion, was painful because she could no longer lift a pot or stand at the stove.

And traveling for business was no longer possible because she couldn't hoist a briefcase. "I was not sleeping at all and barely able to eat," she says. "I had to stop exercising and could not walk more than fifty feet without resting."

As a listener of Dr. Ash's radio show, Pat had always enjoyed his practical, down-to-earth style and his willingness to embrace both traditional and alternative medicine. Pat decided to call him, but couldn't get an appointment. Her boyfriend, who has since become her husband, however, refused to take no for an answer. Instead, he went to Dr. Ash's office, told him her story, and persuaded him to see Pat. "I think he had about twenty-five patients lined up that day," Pat says. "But he cancelled all his appointments and spent the day with me."

Dr. Ash spent hours getting the history of her life. "His first concern was the amount of medicine I was on, which included steroids, blood pressure pills, thyroid pills, pain killers, hormone replacement, sleeping pills, anti-inflammatory pills, and others," Pat says.

Dr. Ash put Pat on a strict diet that eliminated meat, dairy, white flour, nuts, grains, sugar, night shades like eggplant, aged foods including cheese and vinegar, and any foods that were artificial and processed. She also started taking supplements and getting intravenous vitamin drips of vitamin C, sometimes for three hours at a time with the help of a visiting nurse. She also did acupuncture and relaxation therapy.

The alternative therapies made her feel better and put her on the road to recovery. But she still had lapses of severe pain, a lack of strength, and an inability to focus. That's when Dr. Ash introduced her to another doctor, a rheumatologist named Dr. Israel Jaffe.

Dr. Jaffe knew in an instant that Pat had RA. But finding the right mix of medications turned out to be extremely difficult and remains a work in progress. Pat suffered debilitating side effects from methotrexate and experienced little improvement in her symptoms. She's also experimented with Remicade, Enbrel, Arava, and most recently Humira. But whether the current combination of Humira and low-dose methotrexate is working remains to be seen. "It is the last hope for me in this family of products," Pat says.

Despite all these treatment efforts, Pat lives with persistent pain. She continues getting vitamin C injections to strengthen her weak back, and she still takes a cocktail of supplements. She also sees a chiropractor for biweekly adjustments. "I cope with the pain one day at a time," she says.

Having RA has caused Pat enormous stress and created changes for her, both at home and at the office. Not being able to do all that she was accustomed to doing made her frustrated. At home, she had to abandon her passion for cooking and sewing. She also had to scale back the flurry of activity that had become her routine during the Christmas season. Before she was sick, Pat always decorated and cooked for the holidays. With RA, she couldn't hang a wreath or trim her tree without help.

RA also had a significant impact on her work. Early on, her pain was compounded by the stress of trying to hide her condition. "I was challenged to keep my illness from my clients for fear they would see it as a weakness and question my ability to perform or deliver on my work," she says.

To make the adjustments she desperately needed, Pat hired a life coach who helped her learn to approach and do her job differently. Before she got sick, she traveled all over the world for days on end, then came back and headed for the office. Now when she does travel, she makes sure to take days off to rest in between.

She's also become more forthcoming about her condition with clients. "When I'm at a meeting, I have to brace myself to get up from a chair," she says. And her staff is well aware of her limitations. "They understand the situation and know that I do my best to mentor and deliver on my responsibilities," Pat says. "I am very lucky to have my own business. If I need to go, my staff will pick up the ball and run with it. And now after twenty-two years, the business is growing organically."

Not everyone is so sympathetic, however. Because her condition is not obvious to unsuspecting strangers, people have been rude and insensitive. At the grocery store not long ago, a policeman questioned her use of the handicapped parking spot. He demanded to see her disabled person identification card to verify that the placard hanging on her rearview mirror was actually hers.

"I was so upset about the whole thing that I went home without buying my groceries," she says.

Once at a business meeting, she couldn't open a door and was scolded by a woman behind her who pointedly told Pat that she was in the way. Another time, while trying a Pilates class, a woman in the class came over and tried to maneuver Pat, so that she could keep up with the class. "I tried to explain that I couldn't hold myself up on my wrists because I have an arthritic condition," Pat says. "She told me I was slowing everyone else down and disrupting the class."

Upsetting as these incidents are, Pat does understand why people mistake her for someone who is healthy and capable. "I'm small, and I'm in good shape," she says. "So when people look at me, they don't see that I have an arthritic condition. But I'm amazed by how cruel and insensitive people can be."

Not every impact from the disease has been negative, though. Over time, Pat, now fifty-six, has learned to ask for help, to accept her slower reaction time, and to respect her body's need for rest. She has learned that she can no longer do everything she did before, and that the change is not such a bad one. At home and at work, she has learned to let go of things she cannot control and to speak up directly about things that bother her. She has also slowed down, so that she can enjoy more time and closer relationships with her daughter from her first marriage, her new husband, and her three stepchildren.

Overall, life has become much simpler, less hectic, and Pat is pleased with those changes.

"When I look back on my life, I wonder if I appreciated all the blessings I had," she says. "I moved through life so fast that I'm sure I wasn't stopping to smell the roses. I expected such perfection of myself, and I'm sure I put so much pressure on myself that I must have wasted a lot of energy on that effort."

Pat is fairly certain that her RA was triggered by a combination of circumstance, environment, and a familial predisposition toward having the disease.

Shortly before the onset of her symptoms, Pat lost her brother-in-law, who she says was also her best friend and business partner of seventeen years. The devastation of his sudden and unexpected death was compounded by the fact that she now had to manage the business alone and was under undue stress.

Around that same time, she was traveling frequently to mold-infested dairy farms and had just moved into a house with an unexpected mold problem, not knowing that she had a severe allergy to mold. She has since discovered that her cousin has RA, too.

For Pat, finding the two doctors and adopting their dual approach to treatment saved her life. "I would suggest that people consider both traditional and alternative therapies," she says. "It is what has made a difference for me and continues to make it possible for me to work and function and be whole again. The traditional without the alternative is a challenge. And depending on the severity of the disease, the alternative without the traditional may not work hard enough."

CHAPTER ELEVEN ✬

Complications of RA

As a person with RA, you already know about the overwhelming fatigue, the fever, and the general malaise that can accompany your swollen joints. You know about the achiness in your joints, the changes in the appearance of your hands, and the stiffness in your wrists. But because RA is a systemic disease, it can affect other parts of your body as well and cause other complications, some of them rather serious. Your eyes may become drier than usual, your bones may become brittler, and your breathing may become difficult.

Some of these complications are rare and occur only in cases when the disease is severe. But knowing what you might experience will help you remain vigilant.

THE LUNGS

Every day, we take thousands of breaths without giving it a second thought. But in some people who have RA, breathing can become difficult because the disease affects their lungs, causing what is sometimes called rheumatoid lung disease. Rheumatoid lung disease actually refers to several conditions that include pleurisy, pleural effusion, and pulmonary fibrosis.

Pleurisy. This condition occurs in 10 to 20 percent of people with RA. Pleurisy develops when the pleura, the membrane that lines the chest cavity and surrounds each lung, becomes inflamed. If you have pleurisy, you may experience a sharp pain in your chest when you breathe. The pain tends to worsen with coughing, sneezing, moving, or deep breathing. Your doctor may do a chest X-ray or blood tests to determine whether you have pleurisy.

Pleural effusion. Sometimes, pleurisy is accompanied by pleural effusion. This rare complication of RA occurs when excess fluid accumulates between the layers of the pleura. In some cases, there are no symptoms. But some people may have difficulties breathing, shortness of breath, a cough, or a fever. The condition can be detected by X-ray, an ultrasound of the chest, or thoracentesis, the removal of fluid for analysis. Both pleurisy and pleural effusion tend to improve if the underlying condition, in this case RA, improves.

Pulmonary fibrosis. The official name, diffuse interstitial pulmonary fibrosis, refers to a cluster of conditions in which inflammation and scarring of the air sacs, or alveoli, and their supporting structures, the interstitium, decrease lung function. As a result, there is a reduction in the transfer of oxygen from the air to the blood. Symptoms include shortness of breath, a decreased tolerance for activity, and a dry cough. Chest X-rays, pulmonary function tests, blood tests, and CT scans of the chest may be used to diagnose pulmonary fibrosis.

Some patients will develop rheumatoid nodules on their lungs. The nodules are usually harmless and often produce no symptoms. Occasionally the nodules may cause coughing or chest pain. They are usually detected only by X-ray. The nodules may increase in size, disappear spontaneously on their own, or appear in new places as older ones go away. Sometimes, the nodules may need to be removed for biopsy to determine the cause.

In general, complications of the lung are more common in men than in women. Also, not surprisingly, they're more likely to occur in people who smoke. The use of certain medications, such as methotrexate, gold, penicillamine, and cyclophosphamide, also causes a slight increase in the risk for lung problems, though the benefits obtained from the medication usually override that risk. Any difficulties in breathing should be reported to your doctor immediately.

THE BONES

People who have RA are at greater risk of developing osteoporosis, thinning of the bones. Osteoporosis, or porous bone, is a disease characterized by low bone mass and structural deterioration of bone tissue, leading to bone fragility and an increased susceptibility to fractures, especially of the hip, spine, and wrist, although any bone can be affected.

According to the National Osteoporosis Foundation, osteoporosis is a major public health threat for an estimated forty-four million Americans, or 55 percent of the people fifty years of age and older. Approximately ten million individuals in the United States have the disease, and thirty-four million more are estimated to have low bone mass, placing them at increased risk for osteoporosis. If you have RA, your chance of having osteoporosis is significantly increased.

Osteoporosis weakens the bones and puts you at greater risk for fractures, especially in the hips and spine. The inflammation associated with RA appears to play a role in the destruction of bone. Pro-inflammatory cytokines produced in the RA process stimulate a protein called osteoprotegerin, which, in turn, promotes the activity of osteoclasts, a substance that breaks down bone.

Compounding the problem is the use of glucocorticoids, medications that slow the rate of bone formation and interfere with the body's use of calcium and the sex hormones that sustain our bones. According to the American College of Rheumatology, anyone who has taken a glucocorticoid such as prednisone for more than three months is at greater risk for osteoporosis. In addition, the pain of RA may interfere with the ability to perform weight-bearing exercises that help build bone.

Women are naturally at greater risk for osteoporosis than men because they have less bone mass to begin with. The disease is also more common in older people, people who have small bone structure or a history of osteoporosis, and people who smoke, drink a lot of alcohol, or do not eat foods high in calcium and vitamin D. In addition, the disease is more common among people from non-Hispanic white and Asian ethnic backgrounds.

Often, you don't know you have osteoporosis until you break a bone and require an X-ray. But simple tests that measure bone mineral density can tell you before that whether you have osteoporosis.

Unlike some other complications, you can take action to help prevent or at least stave off osteoporosis. To maintain healthy bones, make sure to get enough calcium in your diet. Experts recommend 1,000 milligrams a day for premenopausal women and 1,500 for women who are postmenopausal and not taking estrogen replacement therapy. An eight-ounce serving of milk or yogurt supplies about 300 milligrams of calcium. You should also be sure to get enough vitamin D, either through foods that are fortified or from exposure to the sun. Vitamin D helps the body to absorb calcium. Twenty to thirty minutes of sunlight on your hands or face two or three times a week is generally enough.

Your doctor may also prescribe medications to prevent and treat osteoporosis. Medications such as alendronate (Fosamax), risedronate (Actonel), calcitonin (Calcimar, Miacalcin), raloxifen (Evista), teriparatide (Forteo), and estrogen or hormone replacement therapy all help maintain bone strength.

Finally, avoid smoking and drinking, which can increase your risk for osteoporosis. Do some weight-bearing exercises like walking or bicycling to help your bones stay strong.

THE EYES AND MOUTH

The inflammation that causes the symptoms of RA can sometimes spread to the eyes, causing discomfort, redness, or dryness. Approximately 25 percent of all RA patients will experience some problems with their eyes. Conditions that may result include:

Sjögren's syndrome. When tear glands in the eyes become inflamed, the eyes start producing fewer tears and become uncomfortably dry. Without adequate moisture, they may feel gritty or itchy. You may feel as if you have something in your eye. Inside the mouth, inflammation may occur in the salivary glands, causing excessive dryness.

Dry eyes and mouth may be diagnosed as Sjögren's syndrome. Sjögren comes from the name of a Danish ophthalmologist who described the condition in his doctoral thesis. The condition is worsened by certain medications, dry air, or arid weather conditions. The use of over-the-counter eye lubricants or artificial tears can usually alleviate the problem. If you have dry mouth, talk to your doctor about pilocarpine (Salagen) and cevimeline (Evoxac), medications that stimulate the production of saliva.

If you do have dry mouth, be sure to practice good oral hygiene. A dry mouth promotes tooth decay. Be sure to floss once a day and brush twice a day to eliminate plaque between teeth and on the surface of your teeth. It's also important to see your dentist twice a year for a thorough cleaning and checkup. Approximately one in six patients with RA will experience dry eyes and mouth.

Episcleritis. When inflammation strikes the connective tissue between the conjunctiva—the transparent tissue that covers the outer surface of the eye—and the sclera, known as the episclera, or the white of the eye, you may have episcleritis or scleritis. The condition resembles conjunctivitis, or pink eye, but you usually do not experience a discharge or tearing.

The condition is typically diagnosed by an ophthalmologist using special high-beam equipment. He may prescribe artificial tears for relief. Some patients may also need steroids to reduce inflammation. Left untreated, the condition may cause problems with vision.

Keratitis. People who have RA are more vulnerable to keratitis, an inflammation or irritation of the cornea. The condition is often characterized by a cloudiness or loss of luster in the transparent membrane covering the iris and pupil. Patients may notice pain, blurred vision, sensitivity to light, itching, or watery eyes.

Keratitis varies in severity and usually occurs after the cornea has been injured or penetrated, which allows for bacteria or fungi to enter. In patients with RA, dryness and inflammation make the cornea more vulnerable. Keeping the eyes well-hydrated with artificial tears can reduce the risk.

THE HEART

Cardiovascular disease is the leading cause of death in America, and there's no doubt that RA elevates your risk for developing it. In fact, a 2003 study by researchers at Harvard Medical School found that women who have RA are twice as likely to have a heart attack than women who do not have the disease. The risk is tripled among women who have had RA for ten years or longer.

The link between heart disease and RA is becoming increasingly clear. For one, the inflammation that causes RA is also believed to contribute to atherosclerosis, the buildup of fatty plaque in the arteries and a primary cause of heart attack. High levels of C-reactive protein, a substance released by the body in response to injury or infection, is present in both RA and cardiovascular disease.

At the same time, having RA can cause lifestyle changes that raise your odds for developing heart disease. The swelling, pain, and fatigue of RA can make it difficult for you to get the regular physical activity you need to keep your weight down, lower your blood pressure and cholesterol levels, and improve the function of your heart. In addition, certain medications used to treat RA may increase your risk for heart disease.

RA may also cause other problems in your heart, though heart complications are generally rare. For instance, RA may cause pericarditis, inflammation of the pericardium, which is the thin membrane that surrounds the heart and the roots of the great blood vessels. Once it is inflamed, the action of the pericardium is restricted, causing a sharp, piercing pain over the center or left side of the chest. The pain typically worsens when you're taking a deep breath, and it may also be accompanied by a fever. Treatment is usually with an analgesic or anti-inflammatory medication. If the fluid buildup becomes significant, you may develop pericardial effusion, which may require corticosteroids and, rarely, drainage of the fluid.

THE BLOOD

Consider blood your body's internal transport system, the delivery network of oxygen, nutrients, and other important substances. In people who have RA, the blood may become affected. Here are some of the problems that may occur:

Anemia of chronic disease. Some people who have RA may develop anemia of chronic disease, a deficiency in the number of red blood cells. Anemia affects between one-half and two-thirds of all people with RA. The anemia develops as a result of long-term inflammation, and its severity often mirrors the seriousness of the RA. But when the disease is brought under control, the anemia tends to improve, too.

Iron-deficiency anemia. This condition may result from taking nonsteroidal anti-inflammatory drugs that irritate the stomach lining and cause bleeding. If you develop iron-deficiency anemia, your doctor should try to determine whether the loss of blood is coming from your stomach. You may need to discontinue your NSAIDs and receive treatments to heal your stomach.

Felty's syndrome. Blood problems can also result from another complication of RA, called Felty's syndrome. This relatively rare condition causes an enlarged spleen and a decrease in white blood cells. The spleen is the largest organ in your lymphatic system. A reduction in white blood cells means a decrease in the strength of your immune system, which may make you more vulnerable to infection. You may develop deep sores, or ulcers, on your legs. Felty's syndrome can also cause a decrease in the number of blood platelets, which are critical to your blood's ability to clot. A reduction in blood platelets may lead to excessive bleeding.

Felty's syndrome is rare and usually occurs only if your RA is severe or after you've had the disease for more than ten years. Treatment usually involves taking disease-modifying antirheumatic drugs such as methotrexate. In rare situations, the spleen may need to be removed.

Vasculitis. The blood vessels may experience complications from RA as well. Vasculitis, inflammation of the blood vessels, is a rare complication of RA that may occur when too many antibodies are being produced. When the antibodies stick together, they form clumps known as immune complexes. These complexes may then deposit themselves on the blood vessel walls, causing inflammation and restricting the ability of blood to flow freely.

If vasculitis affects small blood vessels, you may develop skin ulcers. In the area near your fingernails, you may see splinterlike lesions. These skin problems will require vigilant cleansing and care in order to prevent further infection.

Albeit rare, vasculitis can also affect large blood vessels that lead to internal organs. If vasculitis affects blood vessels leading to the nerves, you may experience numbness or weakness. If it affects the intestines, you may experience abdominal pain, bloating, and bloody stools. In the lungs, vasculitis can cause shortness of breath or a cough that produces blood. When the nerves or kidneys are involved, you will need very strong medications like cyclophosphamide to treat the condition and prevent damage.

Raynaud's syndrome. People with RA are vulnerable to Raynaud's syndrome. With Raynaud's, the blood vessels in your hands and feet, or the tips of your nose and ears, go into vasospasms in response to the cold or stress. The vasospasms constrict the blood vessels, dramatically limiting blood supply and causing the fingers or other affected areas to become white and clammy, even blue or purplish. Even something as simple as removing an item from the freezer can trigger a Raynaud's attack. Once you begin warming up your fingers, circulation is restored. Often, the fingers tingle and turn red during the recovery period.

THE NERVES

The body's nervous system is an intricate web of electrical wires and impulses that are activated by the brain, the control center. Whether it's your heart beating or the simple act of opening a drawer, everything we do is governed by our nervous system. In people who have RA, the nerves can become damaged. Inflammation of the blood vessels, or vasculitis, that lead to the nerves is one form of neuropathy. But in some cases, the blood vessels are not involved, and the patient simply develops numbness or a burning sensation.

Patients with RA are also prone to developing entrapment neuropathies. The swelling inside a joint can pinch the nerves beside it. If the swelling or pressure gets bad enough, it will irritate the nerve, sending sensations of pain, numbness, or tingling to the brain and causing a condition called nerve entrapment. When nerve entrapment occurs at the wrist, it is known as carpal tunnel syndrome. Carpal tunnel develops when the median nerve that runs through the wrist becomes compressed as the wrist swells and pressure builds inside the joint. Although the problem is in the wrist, the pain is felt in the thumb, the index finger, and half of the middle finger. If it occurs at the elbow, it is called ulnar nerve entrapment. In that case, you'll feel the pain in your pinky. It is important to have nerve entrapment treated early for best results.

It is important to notify your doctor if you're experiencing numbness and/or tingling. Wrist splints can help reduce the pain of carpal tunnel, as can anti-inflammatory medications or corticosteroid injections in the wrist. In some cases, surgery may be needed to alleviate the pain.

THE SKIN

Approximately a quarter of all people with RA will develop rheumatoid nodules, small bumps beneath the skin that tend to form near joints. These usually harmless nodules are more common among people with positive rheumatoid factor in their blood. But because they are a hallmark of the disease, they are one factor used to diagnose RA.

In most cases, the nodules are painless and moveable. They may become painful if they occur in a location that is frequently traumatized, such as the heel of the foot. In rare instances, they may become so large that they interfere with the functioning of the nearby joint or cause a breakdown of the skin. Though nodules are usually harmless, they do indicate that the RA is rather serious. And for reasons that are poorly understood, methotrexate can sometimes cause an increase in the number of nodules in some patients.

The skin may also be involved if vasculitis occurs. The skin may develop a snakelike appearance and become tender to the touch. In addition, RA may cause the skin to develop large bruises or petechiae, pinpoint dots of blood caused by bleeding into the skin. Any changes in your skin should be brought to the attention of your doctor.

CANCER RISK

In general, people with RA do not have a higher overall risk for cancer and may even have a lesser risk for colon cancer. But people with rheumatoid arthritis are at greater risk for developing lymphoma, a cancer that affects the body's lymphatic system, which together with blood forms the body's immune system. A Swedish study of more than 11,000 RA patients found that the serious inflammation from arthritis contributed to lymphoma risk.

Some experts believe that the use of anti-tumor necrosis factor (TNF) medications may further increase the incidence of lymphoma, but pinpointing that connection has been difficult. Instead, the risk for developing lymphoma may be more closely linked to the severity of RA, and it's those patients with more severe cases of RA who wind up taking anti-TNF drugs.

THE KIDNEYS

Think of the kidneys as the body's filtering system, where toxins enter through tiny blood vessels, are converted into urine, and then are disposed of from the body. In rare cases, your kidneys may be affected by RA. Kidney involvement may be the result of the disease itself or the medications you take to treat it. People who have RA are vulnerable to developing microalbuminuria, a condition in which small amounts of protein appear in the urine. The condition signals that there are changes occurring in the blood vessels of your kidneys and is often the first sign of kidney disease. A Danish study found that RA patients are more likely to have microalbuminuria, and that treatment with gold and penicillamine seems to increase the risk for it.

The chronic inflammation of RA as well as the use of gold, penicillamine, or NSAIDs may also cause a condition called membranous nephropathy, a thickening of the capillary wall inside the kidneys that's caused by inflammation. In addition, the chronic inflammation in RA may cause secondary amyloidosis, in which protein deposits in the kidneys impair kidney function.

THE VOCAL CORD

In some patients, RA may affect the joints inside the vocal cord, called the cricoarytenoid joint, which is located inside the larynx. Often, this complication occurs with no symptoms. But in some people, it may cause hoarseness, difficulty swallowing, a feeling of fullness in the throat, or pain traveling from the throat to the ears. In very severe but rare cases, this inflammation can constrict the airway, making breathing difficult.

A FINAL NOTE

There's no doubt that RA is much more than simply a disease of the joints and that its devastating effects can spread throughout the body. The good news is that advances in the medications used for RA have dramatically improved the prognosis for most patients. Early diagnosis, coupled with early, more aggressive treatment of the disease, has helped slow its progression and stopped the destruction of the joints. With the reduction in inflammation, RA is less likely to spread to other parts of the body, which ultimately lessens your risk for complications.

PROFILE

TERESA

Most people develop arthritis in adulthood, long after they've established careers, married, and started to raise a family. But for Teresa, the disease began in her youth. At fourteen, she was diagnosed with juvenile rheumatoid arthritis (JRA) and warned of how JRA could stunt the growth of her bones. She was also told the disease would subside with age.

As it turns out, the disease did not stunt the development of her bones. But it also didn't go away as she got older. Instead, it got worse. Several doctors were convinced she simply had early-onset RA.

Because it began at such a young age, RA has had profound effects on Teresa's life. A stellar student, she headed for Cornell University in the early 1970s as a theater major with a minor in costume design. But getting around the large and hilly campus was difficult, and the disease was progressing rapidly. Eventually, Teresa could barely walk, much less navigate the stairs that led to her classrooms.

"This was at a time before the Americans with Disabilities Act," she says. "And I didn't have the confidence in myself to speak up."

After attending part-time for a while, Teresa dropped out of Cornell. "It was very hard to go, but I was also relieved by my decision," she says. "I didn't have the stamina to do the work. With RA, your energy is sapped, and you're just overwhelmed."

Teresa headed to New York City and began doing some sewing for theater productions. "It was really hard because I couldn't do much," she says. "Eventually, I had to stop doing the theater work, too." Instead, she spent most of her days going to doctor appointments and seeing her physical therapist.

Through her sister, she met her future husband, Kurt, a cabinet maker, whom Teresa introduces as "her hero." The couple have known each other now for thirty years and been married for twenty-six of those.

Kurt remembers how his wife struggled with RA in New York City and how she tried numerous medications and therapies, including acupuncture. It wasn't until she found a good doctor that her symptoms began to improve, he says. "She became more confident of her abilities."

When the relationship got serious, Kurt accompanied her to a physiatrist, who sat down with the couple to explain the challenges of living with someone with RA. "It was his idea to go," Teresa says. "He really wanted to know about the disease. He saw me taking aspirin all the time and trying all these different medicines. The physiatrist was wonderful and made time after hours to educate him about the disease."

Kurt was undaunted by the challenges, and the couple married soon after. In the meantime, Teresa was growing weary of going to the doctor's office all the time. She was helping her husband with his office work, but spent much of her time as a patient. She knew that if she didn't take action, she could spend the rest of her life in physical therapy. "I wanted to get out of being a sick person," she says. "I wanted to work and to be gainfully employed. And it wasn't like I was going to be crippled if I didn't do physical therapy for a few days."

An evening computer course sparked her interest, and Teresa began thinking about college again. Her strong academic record made her a candidate for Columbia University and New York University. But in the end, she chose Pace University because it was small, accessible, and easily navigated. This time, she enrolled as a math and computer science major.

She kept her ambition in check, knowing from past experience that college would be a challenge. "At first I said, 'I'm just going to get through this semester,'" Teresa recalls. "But then when I got straight As, I said, 'Now, I'm going to get through this next year.'"

While at Pace, Teresa had trouble walking and spent her years there using a cane or a wheelchair. However, she found that ramps intended for wheelchairs were tough to ascend when she was hobbling in on crutches or a cane. Once at the door, she had to get the attention of the person at the front desk, so they could open the door for her.

Teresa hated it. She hated the notion that she had to get the attention of the person on the other side of the door when all she wanted to do was blend in with the other students. "But I realized that if I was quiet and mousy about it, I was never going to get access," she says. "In that case, I could spend my days at home and never get access to anything."

Teresa got in touch with a professor who was the ombudsman for what was then called handicapped issues. She also hooked up with another professor who used crutches and a student who had cerebral palsy. Together, they convinced the facilities department at Pace to give disabled people a card that you could slide into a device, which would then trigger the door to open.

Halfway through her years at Pace, Teresa took some time off to start a family. "I knew that in order to succeed with this disease, I was going to have to give myself a break and just be really patient," she says. She resumed her studies shortly after her daughter was born.

After graduating, Teresa did a stint in the corporate world but didn't like it. She dreamed of working for Bell Labs and doing something more scientific. When she got pregnant with her son, however, she decided she no longer wanted to work full-time. Soon she had two kids, and she wanted more time with her children.

Teresa began toying with the idea of working from home. A friend was proofreading mass-market textbooks, and Teresa began thinking she could do the same for math and computer textbooks. Her first proofreading projects were for McGraw Hill.

Soon, she joined an editors' association and started copyediting, too. The work poured in, and eventually Teresa had to hire another editor to help. In 1991, she started her own editing company, which recently merged with another company.

Over the years, even as her business flourished, Teresa continued dealing with difficulties caused by her RA. She spent years in a wheelchair or walking with a cane or crutches. She had a synovectomy to relieve the pain and swelling in her knee.

Her hands and wrists became increasingly deformed, and she developed ulnar deviation and Boutonniere deformity. She underwent fusion surgery on her wrists and can no longer bend them. She also had extensive hand surgery on her thumb and fingers. The surgeries helped enormously. "The wrist fusions really helped by stabilizing what had become very diseased joints and taking all the pain away," Teresa says. "I have had much more function since the wrist fusions and the hand surgery."

These days, she still experiences the occasional flare from RA. She takes an NSAID every day, along with an occasional Tylenol, but is otherwise free of medications. She relies on assistive devices to help her open jars and special knives for cooking, and asks her family to help with lifting. But she no longer uses a cane or a wheelchair to get around.

Her husband has equipped their house with large handles on every door, her desk drawers, the kitchen cabinets, and her bedroom dresser. "I forget I have all this stuff at home until I'm somewhere else for a while and realize how difficult it is to open doors," she says.

Teresa is well aware of how far she's come since the days she struggled to make it to class at Cornell. Even she is sometimes amazed by her accomplishments. "I used to look at myself as a person with arthritis, a person of disability," she says. "After I had kids, I started thinking of myself as a mom. Now, I see myself as a career woman, and that's really something."

Perhaps most telling of all is the location of her new office: It's up a flight of stairs on the second floor of an old theater. "That would have been unthinkable ten years ago," Teresa says.

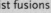

CHAPTER TWELVE ❧

The Emotional Aspects of RA

A chronic disease like rheumatoid arthritis can arouse a range of emotions. You may experience sadness, even depression, over the loss of your physical functioning and mobility. You may be stressed out by the challenges of managing your condition and getting things done. You may be angry that you've been diagnosed with RA even after all your efforts to take care of your health.

Consider all these emotions normal reactions to what is certainly a challenging medical condition. The key is to accept the way you feel, to deal with your feelings, and then to make sure that negative emotions don't interfere with your ability to take care of yourself.

DEPRESSION

Feeling more than a little blue is not uncommon, especially if you have a disease like RA. After all, the disease impacts so many aspects of your life, from getting a good night's sleep to being able to perform your job. But if you develop depression, then your sadness is something more serious that may need medical attention.

Depression is a serious mood disorder that impairs the way you function. An estimated 9.5 percent of the U.S. population—or a staggering nineteen million people—suffer from a depressive illness every year. Left untreated, the disease can ravage your family life, career, and relationships, causing enormous pain and suffering.

Among people with RA, depression is common. Studies have found that people with RA are more likely to be depressed than peers who are not afflicted. In fact, studies in the United Kingdom have found that almost 11 percent of people with RA have had suicidal thoughts.

How can you distinguish the occasional bout of the blues from a case of full-blown depression? It's normal for everyone to feel down on occasion, and having a disease like RA is certainly cause for grief. But according to the National Institute of Mental Health, there are certain telltale signs that indicate you have depression:

- Persistent sad, anxious, or empty mood
- Feelings of hopelessness and pessimism
- Feelings of guilt, worthlessness, and helplessness
- Loss of interest or pleasure in hobbies and activities you once enjoyed, including sex
- Decreased energy, fatigue, and feeling slowed down
- Difficulty concentrating, remembering, or making decisions
- Insomnia, early awakening, or oversleeping
- Appetite changes or fluctuations in weight
- Thoughts of death or suicide, or actual suicide attempts
- Restlessness or irritability

If you're plagued with at least five of these symptoms every day for at least two weeks, and they're beginning to interfere with your daily functioning, consult a medical expert who specializes in depression. Health professionals trained to deal with depression include psychiatrists, psychologists, licensed social workers, psychiatric nurses, and mental health counselors.

Treating Depression

If you determine that you do indeed have depression, you will need treatment. Untreated depression can interfere with your day-to-day functioning and disrupt your ability to care for your arthritis. It can also worsen your pain.

To alleviate your depression, your mental-health professional may prescribe medications, psychotherapy, or a combination of both, depending on your health history and personal preference. Your drug options include:

- **Selective serotonin reuptake inhibitors (SSRIs).** These medications work by blocking the removal of serotonin, a neurotransmitter involved in regulating mood, in the synapses, or gaps between the nerves. Having inadequate amounts of serotonin, as well as other neurotransmitters such as dopamine and norepinephrine, is often the cause of depression. Common SSRIs include fluoxetine (Prozac), paroxetine (Paxil), escitalopram (Lexapro), and sertraline (Zoloft). Possible side effects include jitteryness, headache, nervousness, insomnia, and sexual problems.

- **Tricyclics.** These drugs work by restoring imbalances in the brain that can cause depression. Although initially introduced to treat depression, these medications are also used to reduce the symptoms of panic attacks, post-traumatic stress disorder (PTSD), and obsessive compulsive disorder (OCD). Among the drugs in this category are amitriptyline (Elavil), clomipramine (Anafranil), imipramine pamoate (Tofranil PM), and nortriptyline (Aventyl). These medications generally have more side effects than the SSRIs, including dry mouth, constipation, and blurred vision.

- **Monoamine oxidase inhibitors (MAOIs).** Strict dietary requirements while taking these medications have made them a less popular option than other antidepressants. If taken with certain cheeses and wines that contain a substance called tyramine, MAOIs can cause extremely high blood pressure. Taking them with nasal decongestants can cause similar problems. The drugs in this category are also used to treat panic disorder, social phobia, PTSD, and sometimes OCD. Drugs in this class are isoarboxazid (Marplan), phenelzine (Nardil), and tranylcypromine (Parnate).

• **Other antidepressants.** Some drugs used to treat depression don't share the same chemical structure with one another but have the same goal of stabilizing the chemicals in the brain, namely serotonin, norepinephrine, and dopamine. Drugs in this loosely organized category include buproprion (Wellbutrin), venlafaxine (Effexor), and mirtazapine (Remeron). Lithium, another drug in this category, is more commonly used to treat manic-depressive symptoms.

Using Psychotherapy

If taking another medication is unappealing to you, you may want to consider psychotherapy, a strategy for overcoming depression that involves talking. Discussing your depression with a trained therapist can help you overcome your feelings of intense sadness. A type of therapy known as cognitive-behavioral therapy works by changing the way the patient thinks and behaves in order to reduce depression. If the source of the depression involves other people, you may be inclined to try interpersonal therapy.

STRESS

Stress is an inescapable reality of life. We experience stress in our relationships with loved ones, in our jobs, and in our neighborhoods and communities. We feel stress when we drive through traffic, stand in long lines, and do our errands. We even experience stress during joyous times, such as the holidays, vacations, or the start of a new job we've always wanted.

Living with a chronic disease creates a kind of stress unlike any other, and RA can cause worries you never before experienced. You worry about how you'll manage day-to-day tasks that once seemed so simple, like cooking a meal or cleaning your house. You fret about the prospect of not being able to perform your job and becoming disabled. You worry about the medications you're taking and whether they'll work this time. You become anxious as you contemplate your future.

The stress of RA can be overwhelming, especially if you're having difficulty bringing the disease under control. But managing your stress is more important than ever to your health. In fact, experts suspect that RA can be triggered by stress just as stress can cause high blood pressure or high cholesterol.

How Stress Affects the Body

Imagine yourself lying in your bed alone when you suddenly hear someone entering your house through the back door. All senses go into high alert as you sit up in bed, your heart racing. These external responses are the result of internal changes that begin inside the brain, where the hypothalamus releases corticotropin-releasing hormone (CRH). In turn, CRH triggers the release of norepinephrine, epinephrine, and cortisol, three hormones that work together to help the body brace itself to fight or flee, by temporarily improving strength and agility, bolstering concentration and reaction time, and mobilizing reserves of fat and carbohydrates for immediate energy. If the person breaking into your house suddenly comes into your bedroom, you've braced yourself for a fight.

Now imagine that you realize the noise is simply coming from your next-door neighbor's house, and you realize he's coming home late. The threat disappears, your heart rates slows, and you feel calmer. Inside your body, while the other hormones have stopped exerting their effects, cortisol remains, acting on your brain to halt the production of CRH in order to stop the stress response.

Under normal circumstances, stress and the secretion of cortisol is a good thing; cortisol is a vital hormone that is responsible for the metabolism of carbohydrates, proteins, and fats, and regulation of the immune system. The problem occurs when stress is chronic, as it is when you're living with a chronic disease like RA. Living with chronic stress keeps cortisol levels elevated, leaving your body in a perpetual state of fight-or-flight, even when there is nothing to run from and your body isn't moving. These high levels of cortisol can weaken your immune system, which is already challenged by RA, and promote weight gain, which can increase the burden on your joints. And if you're feeling helpless, you'll create a vicious cycle of unabated stress.

Taming the Stress Monster

RA creates stress because it involves change—changes in the way you spend your time, in the way you perform certain tasks, possibly even in the way you get out of bed in the morning. The fact that the disease is so unpredictable only exacerbates your stress, especially if you're the type of person who ruminates about the future. And if your condition frequently fluctuates or you're having trouble pinning down the right mix of medications, you'll be dealing with constant adjustments that also cause stress.

In people who have RA, stress causes additional pain. It can make it hard for you to get the sleep you desperately need, even as it creates more fatigue. You may also have reduced functioning of your immune system, high blood pressure, and an increased heart rate.

Taking control over your stress, or stress management, is important for your health because it decreases pain and depression. A

2000 study published in *Arthritis Care Research* attributed the positive effects of stress management to improvements in self-efficacy—the belief that you can perform a specific behavior or task in the future—more confidence in your ability to manage pain, and the sense that you have more control over your arthritis. Participating in a formal stress management program is one way to lessen your stress. But there are also some strategies you can use in your daily life to help you get a handle on stress:

- **Set reasonable goals.** Aiming for goals that are beyond your reach will only cause frustration and angst. So keep your plans within reason and certainly within reach. Ask yourself if you can really accomplish what you're planning. For instance, you may have been able to clean your entire house on a Saturday morning in the days before you were sick. But now that you have a chronic disease, it might be more realistic to simply try to clean just a room or two at a time.
- **Stop worrying about things you can't control.** As you well know, many things in life are out of your control, and RA is one of them. Flares are often unpredictable, the effects of a medication may seem like a mystery, and the day-to-day rhythm of your pain may vary. So stop worrying about them. Instead, focus on what you're dealing with in the moment. That brings up the next tip.
- **Focus on the present.** Rather than worrying about things you did in the past or the course of your disease in the future, put your energies into the present. Fretting about what's done or what's to come can cause needless worry and anxiety that heighten stress levels.
- **Exchange negative thoughts for positive ones.** It isn't always easy to change the way you think, but establishing a

more positive perspective can help reduce your stress. So if you're unhappy with your inability to keep a clean house because of your arthritis, focus on the things you do achieve during a busy day.

• **Establish clear priorities.** Working the annual church bazaar may have been important to you when you were healthy, and it was probably easily done. But having a chronic disease like RA might mean you need to scale back and put your energies into things that are of more importance to you, like spending time with your children.

• **Make time for exercise.** Physical activity not only releases feel-good endorphins; it also distracts you from stressful thoughts and worries. And exercise helps you gain more physical strength and control over RA.

• **Devote some time to relaxation.** Try deep breathing or meditation, which can help lessen the impact of stress. These mental exercises use the mind to settle the body. You might also consider spending time in nature, doing yoga, or writing down your feelings in a journal.

• **Learn to expect the unexpected.** No, you don't know when your aches will worsen or when a blissful spell of remission will turn into a disruptive flare. But if you develop the mind-set that RA is filled with unexpected, unpredictable turns, any changes in your condition will be less surprising and less disturbing.

• **Get professional help, if necessary.** If you have tried to take control of your stress and still find yourself overwhelmed, it might be time to get help from a mental health professional. You might need to take more aggressive action to manage your stress. Prolonged stress can have a negative impact on RA, so it's important to gain some control over it.

ANGER

It's normal to feel angry that you have RA. After all, you did nothing to bring on this condition. In fact, you may have even been the pillar of good health, someone who didn't smoke or drink, ate well, and exercised regularly.

Now that you've been diagnosed with a chronic disease that's causing immense pain, you're furious and possibly asking, "Why me?" You're angry that you have so many doctor's appointments, need to take so many medications, and are missing out on simple pleasures that have become hard to do.

Getting over your anger isn't easy and may take time. But not getting rid of it can take its toll on your condition. Anger can disturb your sleep, exacerbate your pain, and interfere with your ability to take care of yourself. It also saps your already compromised energy levels.

That's why it's important to acknowledge your anger and then to move on. Here are some ways to do that:

- **Pinpoint the source of your anger**. Are you mad because you can't do all the things you used to do? That you're overwhelmed with fatigue? Do you feel helpless? Identify the cause of your anger and try to work on that. You may need to adjust your expectations (see below), create new priorities, and set more realistic goals.
- **Discuss your anger.** Whether you talk to a close friend or a professional counselor, venting about your anger can help reduce it. Your friend or counselor may be able to shed new light on your situation and help you overcome your anger.
- **Develop realistic expectations.** Before you had RA, you could go to the gym every morning, work all day, and then head out and do errands in the evening. These days, you feel as if you can't even get out of bed. Rather than

dwell on what you used to do, create new expectations of yourself. Go to the gym at lunchtime twice a week, or do errands on weekends only. By keeping your expectations realistic and attainable, you'll build your sense of competence and rein in frustration.

- **Channel your anger into positive actions.** Rather than devoting too much energy to feeling mad, try putting your energy into taking positive action. Fed up that you can't cook the way you used to? Think of it as a challenge to find new and simpler recipes. Can't do all the jogging you used to enjoy? Consider it an opportunity to take up a different exercise like yoga.

MIND-BODY TECHNIQUES FOR COPING

The connection between your mind and your body is a powerful one. A 2002 study by researchers at the National Center for Complementary and Alternative Medicine found that mind-body therapies such as progressive muscle relaxation, biofeedback, stress management, and cognitive-behavioral therapy can have significant positive effects on several aspects of RA.

Levels of pain, the ability to function, and joint tenderness all improved with the use of these mind-body techniques. The researchers also saw improvements in depression, coping, and feelings of helplessness. The therapies offered the greatest benefit to RA patients who were recently diagnosed. Over time, the benefits were most pronounced in managing depression and easing the pain of tender joints. We've already explored strategies for stress management, but let's take a closer look at these other mind-body techniques.

Progressive Muscle Relaxation

In 1929, a psychologist from Chicago named Edward Jacobson detailed a technique called progressive muscle relaxation and noted that it is physically impossible to feel pain if the muscles in our bodies are completely relaxed.

Mastering progressive muscle relaxation, however, takes practice. Here's how to do it:

- Locate a quiet place and get into a comfortable position.
- Close your eyes.
- Begin by tensing up your toes for five seconds. Then relax them. Notice the different sensation between tensing and relaxing.
- Progressively move up your body, alternating between tensing, or clenching, and relaxing.
- Continue all the way up to your head.

Biofeedback

The ability to control our autonomic body functions is the premise behind biofeedback. Using imagery or relaxation, you can learn how to control functions like breathing, heart rate, blood pressure, skin temperature, and muscle tension.

The procedure is done using electrodes and monitoring equipment that both you and the trained practitioner can see. While the practitioner describes stressful situations and then guides you through relaxation techniques, you observe the information on the monitor and see how your heart rate, blood pressure, and other functions change in response to being stressed or relaxed. The information is therefore fed back to you, giving you the mental power to regulate and change these body functions.

Mastering biofeedback can make you feel more relaxed and give you the power to treat your own arthritis pain. The technique is also used to treat high blood pressure, migraine headaches, and urinary incontinence, among other conditions.

Cognitive-Behavioral Therapy

With cognitive-behavioral therapy (CBT), the goal is to change the way you think and behave in order to minimize your stress and anxiety. Changing the way you think can affect your physical health. In terms of RA, the goal of cognitive-behavioral therapy is to influence the way you think about your symptoms and your behavior toward that pain.

CBT combines two kinds of psychotherapy: cognitive therapy and behavior therapy. Cognitive therapy teaches you how certain thought patterns may be playing a role in causing your symptoms. For instance, you may have distorted thoughts about your condition, like "Now I'll never be able to garden again," which can cause you anxiety and depression.

Behavior therapy helps you weaken the link between troublesome situations and your reactions to them. For instance, if you typically react to a flare with rage, your therapist will work with you to change that reaction to one that is more positive. It also teaches you how to calm your mind and body, so you can think more clearly and make better decisions. In some ways, CBT is likened to education, coaching, or tutoring.

STAYING HAPPY

These days, it might not be easy for you to feel happy. You've lost the ability to do things you enjoy. Your body is wracked with pain. Sleep is elusive, broken, and fitful. On top of that, you're dealing with an endless number of visits to doctors, trying to keep track of numerous medications, and fretting about the course of your illness.

No doubt, trying to sustain a positive outlook in the face of an illness like RA is difficult. But trying to remain positive is important to your health and may even shape your prognosis. Feeling happy can enhance your immune system and helps ensure that you will engage in healthy behaviors that can alleviate your symptoms.

So how do you stay positive when you're feeling so lousy?

- **Steer clear of distorted thinking.** Avoid persistent negative thinking that can make you feel bad. Don't turn every little event into a major catastrophe. Look for ways to reframe an event and modify the way you view it.
- **Look for deeper meaning.** Whether it's organized religion or deepened spirituality, faith and prayer can be beneficial in helping you cope with RA. Putting your faith in a higher power can help you focus on what's truly important in life.
- **Seek out the company of other people.** It's impossible to handle the emotional rigors of RA alone, so make sure to spend time with people you care about. If you avoid people for fear of unsolicited advice or questions, you will only create greater feelings of isolation and loneliness, and raise your risk for depression.
- **Try to do something you enjoy every day.** Dig up an old movie you loved as a child. Call a friend you haven't spoken to in years. Listen to music you enjoy. Giving some attention to life's pleasurable experiences will help you reduce the negative emotions you feel.

PROFILE

TAMARA

Because Tamara was just six years old when she first began developing arthritis, her parents thought for sure she was simply suffering from the flu or experiencing growing pains. But when her condition deteriorated, her parents took her to an urban hospital, where she was diagnosed with juvenile rheumatoid arthritis (JRA).

Many children who suffer from JRA get relief over time. Tamara did not. Instead, her pain persisted. Today, at thirty-three, Tamara is convinced she simply had juvenile onset rheumatoid arthritis.

As a child with arthritis, Tamara was terribly frightened, especially when the initial diagnosis led to a two-week stay in the hospital. "I was so young that I don't really have memories of those first few days," she says. "I do remember being in the hospital and being very scared. It was probably the first time not sleeping in my own bed, and I was in the city, away from my family. It was an extremely painful and scary time, and I tear up now even thinking about it. It was the start of my feeling different."

Tamara's life quickly became a series of medical tests, physical therapy, and medications. Twice a week, she left class to receive physical therapy in the city. "The other kids thought I was so lucky, and that I was receiving special treatment," Tamara recalls. Later on, it became apparent that Tamara had a great deal of discomfort. She wore a neck brace and hand splints, but was still forced to play sports such as volleyball in gym class.

At college, Tamara struggled to keep up with the other students. "University was difficult in the sense that I had to be quite mobile to make it from one class in one building to the next within ten minutes," she says. "And after sitting still for sometimes ninety minutes, I would become stiff and would struggle to make it to my next class on time. I was also working to pay my way through college and was just exhausted." She earned her college tuition by appearing in television commercials, a job that honed her love for working in media—a love that prompted her to abandon her plans for law school.

Over the years, however, Tamara built up a reserve of strength and sheer willpower that has become her greatest ally in the struggle against RA. She has produced documentaries for TV and appeared as an on-air features and news reporter. She has also been published in magazines and newspapers. Today, as a self-described workaholic, Tamara runs her own freelance business, dabbling in different media. Having RA, she says, has been the greatest factor in her life and has shaped her personality and work ethic.

Tamara is seriously involved with a man she'd like to marry and is in discussions with her doctors about having children someday. "I am just about the most driven, biggest workaholic I have ever known," she says. "I have a whole list of things to accomplish, and though it is so difficult—more than I can really explain some days—I just grit my teeth and push ahead. I am proud of my strength of will and mind, even if I have a weak body. I use that to fuel me through the pain, stiffness, and exhaustion that this disease brings. I am also an incredible fighter and refuse to let this disease get the best of me."

Willpower has been essential to Tamara, who has had little luck with medications. She has tried all kinds of nonsteroidal anti-inflammatory medications and disease-modifying antirheumatic drugs. She has also experimented with complementary therapies such as magnets, supplements, and naturopathy. "I haven't had much luck with any of them," she says. The only one that worked at all was Enbrel, but a fever and chest infection forced her off that medication. Until recently, she was also on Vioxx. "I was told to use Bextra, but I am concerned that it is in the same COX-2 classification as Vioxx and so am not prepared to take it right now." As a result, she currently takes no medication at all.

The lack of treatment, however, does come with a price. "I recently had what I would say was the very worst day with this disease that I've ever had," she confides. "I coped by doing what I always do—gritting my teeth and telling myself, 'You are the toughest woman in the world' and allowing myself thirty minutes of self-pity. Then I nurtured myself and took a day off from work and worries."

She manages her disease with regular swimming, hot baths, and visits to a massage therapist. "I am easier on myself if I need to sleep in or need to have a rest," she says. "I try to schedule only a few errands at a time per day and ask that people in my life be more lenient about appointments and dates with me in case I'm running late. I have recently decided to move about 80 percent of my work to my home, so I can work during my high-energy periods."

Tamara also gives talks to school children, college kids, and med students about her condition, and works hard to dispel a key myth of arthritis: that it's strictly a disease of the elderly. "I once had a lady say to me, 'You can't have arthritis, you're too young!'" she recalls. "She said it like she didn't believe me and was trying to convince me otherwise."

She also likes to educate people who think arthritis—namely osteoarthritis—is an inevitable part of aging. "It's not, and there is so much that can be done to prevent it," she says. "It's important to tell people they should indeed take care of themselves now."

For people who have had the misfortune of developing RA, Tamara stresses the importance of getting educated and learning about the different medications and surgical options. "Do not let the only information you have about the disease be what you get from your doctor," she says. "Get a specialist, and if you're not comfortable with him or her, get another one."

It's also important to surround yourself with a team of professionals that includes a nutritionist and physical therapist. "That way you learn as early as possible the right ways of doing things to minimize the damage to your joints," she says.

Tamara also advises people to adhere to a careful balance of rest and exercise and to be completely honest about what they need with the people around them. "When I buy a bottle of water, I always ask the salesclerk to open the bottle for me," she says. "I have no qualms about asking for help."

Most important, she says, respect the pain you feel. "Understand that it's your body's way of telling you you're hurting something," she says.

CHAPTER THIRTEEN ❧

Getting the Support You Need

Having a chronic disease may feel lonely at times. Others around you may have a difficult time understanding your pain, especially if you look healthy. Your children may not be old enough to comprehend the challenges you face. Your spouse may be overwhelmed, even frightened, by the prospect of spending his life with someone who has a serious disease like RA. As a result, you may feel isolated and alone.

That's why it's important to find or create the support you need. Whether it's a preexisting relationship, say, with a spouse, or a new one with a support group, creating a strong network of social support is important to you and your health. It may help buffer you from the pain of an intense flare-up. It can lift up your spirits on days when you're feeling down. It can help you shift your attention and energies elsewhere. A solid support network offers a palliative that no pharmaceutical can ever deliver.

MAINTAINING INTIMACY

Before you had RA, you probably experienced ups and downs in your marriage or intimate relationships. That's normal. Now that you have RA, your relationship may be more challenged and strained. Sex may be difficult, even painful, if not impossible during a difficult flare-up. Fatigue may sap your energy and limit your enthusiasm for even the simplest activities. The attention you give to managing your condition may interfere with the attention you normally devote to your relationship.

Enduring a bad flare or the challenges of trying a new medication takes enormous patience. If you're lucky, your partner will make an effort to understand what you are experiencing and ask how he or she can help. You can help by educating your partner about the disease and keeping the lines of communication wide open. It can also help to bring your partner to an appointment with your doctor. Not only will your partner develop a better understanding of your disease, but your partner may become better equipped to help you make decisions about it.

Don't forget, too: Your partner is coming to terms with RA as well. He or she may be uncertain of how to approach you. Should he offer help? Should she give you advice? Should he talk about your condition at all or act as if nothing were any different?

The direction of your relationship should rest with you. After all, you are the one confronting the pain, fatigue, and limitations of RA. Only you can tell your partner what it is you want from him and what you need. Whether it's asking your partner to handle the bills from now on or expressing your concern over a lack of intimacy, voicing your concerns to your partner is more critical now than ever. If you don't want him to offer you advice, tell him so. If you'd rather he not discuss your condition with his friends, let him know that. Don't expect that sheer love will produce the kind of understanding you need. You have to speak up and make your voice heard.

SAY WHAT YOU MEAN

Some people may have a hard time expressing their feelings. Others may have difficulty asking for help. Still others may know what they want to say, but have a hard time putting it into a clear message.

Having RA means you'll need to hone your communication skills. If friends want you to join them on an outing you really have no energy for, you need to say so rather than go along out of obligation. If your boss expects you to stay late, but you're too tired and achy, you'll need to let him know and work out an alternative. When your kids are screaming for you to take them somewhere and you can't muster the strength, you have to tell them that you simply can't do it. Don't expect others to be mind readers.

Some people have a difficult time asking for help, but when you have a disease like RA, you will need help from others, especially loved ones. Get in the habit of asking directly for what you want, without laying on a guilt trip, playing the martyr, or antagonizing the recipient of your message. The key is to describe exactly what you need and what you expect from the other person. And to ensure you get the help you want, toss in some appreciation for the other person's efforts. A little charm goes a long way when it comes to asking for help.

SEX AND RA

One of the most important forums for open communication is in the bedroom, where RA is bound to have an impact. Having sex may become extremely difficult for people who have RA. The stress of the illness can easily sabotage desire. You may feel too tired or achy for sex. Or you may feel nervous about the physical challenges sex might cause or embarrassed by the appearance of your joints. Positions that were once pleasurable are now painful, even impossible.

To sustain an active sex life, keep your lines of communication open. Explore different positions for having sex. Do not have sex when you're in the throes of pain since that may only build resentment and disrupt the relationship.

Remember, keeping the intimacy alive in a relationship doesn't have to be simply about sex. The key is to spend time doing things together that forge intimacy, like snuggling on a couch or holding hands while taking a walk. If you have the energy and desire for sex, then by all means, indulge. Orgasms release feel-good endorphins that can help temporarily distract you from the pain of RA. Just remember that it probably won't look like the kind of passion we see on television.

PARENTING WITH RA

Keeping up with your kids may become extremely difficult when you have RA. You may not be able to do as much as you could before you got sick. And the fluctuating nature of the disease makes it hard to give your children the structure and consistency they need.

If your children are old enough, tell them you have RA in terms they can understand. Let them know that there will be days when you'll be in more pain than others, and that there may be activities you can no longer do. Encourage them to discuss how they feel about your illness, so they have a place to vent any frustrations they might have. And don't be hesitant to ask them for help, if they're old enough to perform chores. The additional responsibilities will even help foster their sense of responsibility.

Once your kids start forming friendships, don't hesitate to enlist the help of other parents if you're having difficulty getting your kids to parties and activities. In return, offer to host a homework session or some other activity that is less physically taxing. Again, the key is to speak up and communicate your needs. Don't sit back and expect that people will offer, even if they know you have RA. Only you know the pain and difficulties you're experiencing.

Whatever you do, eliminate the guilt that comes with not being able to be the parent you might have thought you'd be. Your children will sense your guilt and may even use it to manipulate you. Keep in mind that no one, not even a healthy person, is the perfect parent. If you look around closely, you'll see that parenting poses challenges for everyone. Yours just happens to be RA.

STAYING SOCIAL

In the midst of a bad flare-up, you may want little to do with the outside world, preferring instead to hide inside your house. But staying isolated isn't so good for your health. That's why you need friendships that nourish your spirit. You need to surround yourself with friends who are willing to listen to your concerns and feelings, and who will give you encouragement and hope when you need it. You need friends who will offer advice when you need it, but who will stay silent when you don't.

On the other hand, you do not need friends who minimize your condition or who make you feel you must put on a cheerful front, no matter how you really feel. Steer clear of people who are uncomfortable discussing your condition, or who give you excessive pity. These types of people are more likely to make you feel bad about yourself.

The goal is to be selective about how you spend your social time, especially since it has now become more limited and precious. Devote your time and energy to being with people who offer you the support and encouragement you need, who bring you true joy in their presence. Avoid those who sap your energy and make you feel bad.

FORMAL SUPPORT GROUPS

Getting together with other people who are also experiencing RA can help tremendously, so long as the get-togethers aren't focused on complaining. But where, you wonder, do you find these support groups?

Start by asking your doctor if he knows of any. Some practices may even assemble a support group so patients have a forum for sharing ideas. The Arthritis Foundation also offers several different support groups around the country. Among their offerings are the Arthritis Self-Help Course (ASHC), Arthritis Basics for Change (ABC), and EDIT RA, or the Early Diagnosis, Intervention, and Treatment of Rheumatoid Arthritis programs. By going to their Web site at www.arthritis.org and searching for these programs, you can find one in your area. You can also find them by calling a chapter of the Arthritis Foundation near you.

Support is also available on the Internet. Typing in the phrase "rheumatoid arthritis and support groups" produces more than 300,000 hits on Google. Web sites like webmd.com, about.com, and yahoo.com all feature forums, chat rooms, and message boards where you can go online and find others who are living with RA.

FINAL TIPS

Building up a network of strong social support is important for people with RA. Do so wisely, and your support network will buffer you against some of your most difficult periods with RA. Do it badly, and you may wind up with unnecessary stress. Here are some tips:

- **Be selective about everything.** Don't waste time going to a doctor whose bedside manner makes you cringe. Avoid wasting time going to meetings for organizations that no longer mean anything to you. Instead, focus your time and energy on people and events that truly matter. You don't have the energy to spare.
- **Choose your friends wisely.** Chances are, RA has cut back the amount of time you can devote to being with friends. That's why it's important to choose your friends wisely. Look for people who are willing to listen to you when

you need a friendly ear, but who are not overly solicitous of your problems. Surround yourself with kind, caring people, and avoid those who irritate and annoy you. In other words, give time to the people who matter most.

• **Speak up.** In any relationship, be sure to speak your mind. Whether you are troubled by something your doctor has done, are angry at your spouse for not helping with chores, or don't have the energy to attend a friend's baby shower, it's important for you to express yourself. Don't harbor bad feelings that will only cause you undue stress. Remember, stress can exacerbate your pain.

PROFILE

RICK AND CAROL EUSTICE

Had it not been for modern technology and rheumatoid arthritis, it's safe to say that Rick and Carol Eustice might never have met.

The couple became acquainted online in September 1995, when Rick logged on to Carol's chat room on America Online. At the time, Rick lived in California and Carol in Ohio. "We became fast friends," Carol says. "Rick flew to Ohio to meet me in person in May 1996. Our relationship grew gradually, and we realized we had more in common and [more] to share than just RA. We were married in 1997."

By the time they married, both had been living with RA for many years. Carol, who is now forty-nine, was diagnosed in 1974 at the age of nineteen. "My first symptoms occurred when I was walking down some steps at college, and it felt unlike anything I'd ever felt before," she says. "I felt intense pain and weakness in my legs. I went to the doctor, who said I had water on my knee. He drained it and gave me a cortisone shot. But we repeated that procedure four times, two weeks apart, because it kept coming back."

Thinking it was a sports injury, Carol's doctor sent her to see an orthopedic surgeon. X-rays revealed severe joint damage, but laboratory tests of her blood did not show that she had RA. Carol was sent home and told to take eight aspirins a day. "With each pill I swallowed, I also swallowed some hope that this would end soon," she says.

The end, as she says, never came. Instead, the pain intensified and traveled from the left side of her body to the right. Soon all her joints were showing damage, enough damage for her doctor to diagnose her with RA.

The effect on her life was overwhelming. "One day I had no pain, and the next I was facing severe chronic pain," Carol says. "Living with chronic pain changes your mind-set. Whatever goals you have and whatever you are working towards becomes framed by the pain, meaning you have to try to minimize the interference of RA even as you try to get through life, achieve your goals, and build a future."

At first, Carol admits she was in denial. "In my mind, RA was never going to stop me," she says. In fact, when she had her first surgery, a hip re-placement at age twenty-five, she was sure it would be the only surgery she'd ever have.

Her optimism was cut short by the reality of RA, and eventually, the dis-ease did disrupt her plans. She was forced to cut back her hours at her job as a registered medical technologist—a job she'd done for sixteen years—and eventually had to quit and apply for disability. She also went on to have eleven more surgeries, including left and right hip replacements and revisions, knee replacements, and ankle fusions. "Each resulted in 100 percent pain relief for me, but some loss of [range of] motion," she says.

It became apparent that Carol had to adjust her life to fit her new circum-stances. "The physical changes in me were making me into someone different than I had been," she writes on her Web site at arthritis.about.com. "I deter-mined that I needed the mental changes to correlate with the physical changes. I needed not to view the changes in me as a loss but rather as a trans-formation. Arthritis had not destroyed my life, but it had changed it. The focus had to shift from what I had lost to what I still had."

Some changes were simple ones, like moving things from the top shelf to a lower shelf and reorganizing her kitchen, so frequently used things were more accessible. She started wearing slip-on shoes instead of high heels or shoes that required tying. She gave up wearing button-up blouses in favor of pullovers. She cut her hair into a style that was more manageable. She also gave up tennis, which she loved to play.

In May 1995, Carol took her career in a new direction when she started an online chat group on America Online. Two years later, she was asked to be the editor and content producer for a Web site about arthritis. "I've been able to turn my life experience into something that helps other people and helps me at the same time," she says. "It's a win-win. I can work from home, on my own schedule, and within my limitations."

Rick, now forty-three, was diagnosed with RA in 1988, shortly before his twenty-seventh birthday. He was at the peak of his career as a restaurant manager, real estate investor, and part-time tax accountant during tax season. He was also a father of two young boys.

He still remembers one of his first bouts of pain: He was in the middle of installing linoleum, when he stood up and felt intense pain in his hip. "I thought I had injured myself," Rick says. "I went to the doctor, but he found no evidence of injury."

A few months later, Rick developed what he thought was a ganglion cyst on his wrist. The hand went numb, and Rick went to a hand specialist, who told him it was a rheumatoid nodule. Though he did not diagnose Rick with RA, he strongly suspected it and referred Rick to a rheumatologist.

While waiting for the day of his appointment, Rick did a lot of self-treatment to relieve the pain, which was initially mild. He took over-the-counter pain remedies, applied arthritis creams, and took hot showers. He attributed his aches and pains to stress and working too hard.

When Rick went to see the rheumatologist, he was shocked to learn he had RA. "I immediately thought, as most people do, 'Arthritis? Isn't that an old person's disease?'"

Although it wasn't that long ago, doctors at the time were still treating RA rather conservatively. Rick began by taking nonsteroidal anti-inflammatory medications. It wasn't until a few years later that he was given methotrexate and a low dose of steroids.

The disease magnified the problems in his first marriage, and he and his first wife eventually divorced. He was also compelled to change his career course. "I was forced to end my management career, phase myself out of real estate investing, and focus more on my accounting background," he says.

To help him cope, Rick got involved in volunteer work. He cofounded a local support group for young people with arthritis, volunteered as a camp counselor at a summer camp for kids with arthritis, and got involved with the Arthritis Foundation.

In the summer of 1995, he went on the Internet and began building friendships with other people who had RA. It was then that he met Carol and became the cohost of the weekly chats on America Online.

"In May 1996, we met in person," he writes on the arthritis.about.com Web site. "I lived in southern California. She lived in Ohio. Carol was as beautiful and caring in real life as she was in cyberland. Carol relocated to southern California. Our relationship grew, and we truly turned out to be soul mates. In May 1997, we married and became Mr. and Mrs. 'RA' Eustice."

Together, the couple confronted the challenges of RA, which only heightened. For instance, when Carol had her left ankle fused, she developed sepsis, a serious infection of the blood that required a prolonged hospital stay. She underwent a procedure called debridement, which is the removal of nonliving tissue in pressure ulcers, burns, and wounds, done to speed healing, and several weeks of intravenous antibiotic treatment. A couple years later, when Rick had his right foot fused, he developed a staph infection, which required months of antibiotic treatment, debridement, and wound care.

Shortly after the couple relocated to Nevada, Carol had surgical revision of her right hip. During the recovery, she developed an infection. Near the end of her recovery, Rick began experiencing severe swelling in his feet and legs, and problems in his back and spine began impeding his ability to walk. At the hospital, he learned he had pericarditis, a rare complication of RA that involves the buildup of fluid around the heart. Doctors had to drain the fluid from his chest.

But when he got home, his condition did not improve. As it turns out, Rick had developed a staph infection during his stay in the hospital. Doctors had to do another debridement in his chest in order to remove the infection. The healing took considerably longer than expected. Rick spent weeks lying in the hospital, hallucinating and unable to even push the button for help. He lost ninety pounds, and his arms were black and blue from months of using an IV for the antibiotics. "At times, I hesitate to admit, I laid there alone at night in my diaper wondering just how long it could last and how bad it would get," Rick recalls.

Rick finally returned home in April 2002. The infection had taken a terrible toll, and he immediately began physical and occupational therapy to regain his function and mobility. He underwent cataract surgery to repair the damage to his eyes caused by the high-dose steroid treatments during his hospital stay. He also had a synovectomy and tendon transfer done on his wrist.

Gradually, he began to improve. By late 2003, Rick stopped using a platform walker and started walking with a cane. "I have been fighting my way back from this epic illness for over three years now. The toll on me at times was tremendous, but it wasn't only on me—it was on Carol, on my sons, on my other close family and friends, too," he says.

Carol's support was critical to Rick's recovery. "When I finally made it home, Carol was my primary caregiver, though I really prefer the word *share-giving*," Rick says. "She did everything she knew how to do for me. Most important, I drew from her love and inner strength to sustain my own and get me back into our life together."

Being married to someone who has the same disease you do has had many advantages, the couple agrees. "It is truly comforting to have a partner with a unique understanding of RA, and solid support comes with that understanding," Carol says. "We're a team in every way. We get into a bit of a bind only if both of us are sick at the same time. I don't mean aches and pains at the same time. That's a given. If both of us need surgery or are unable to drive at the same time, it can get complicated."

Rick agrees. "Carol and I are a team," he says. "We share everything and do everything together."

On top of sharing a life and a home, they share a group of internal medicine doctors and orthopedic surgeons. "We share a love of reading, music, socializing with family and friends, and a zest for living life within our limitations," Rick says. Rick also assists Carol with writing the about.com Web site. Together, they say, they have forty-five years of experience with the disease.

Not surprisingly, they both have plenty of advice for people who are just beginning their struggles with RA. Team up with the best rheumatologist possible, they advise. Avoid the negative impact of being around people who don't understand you. Give yourself the chance to mourn what the disease has cost you, without wallowing in depression. Learn as much as you can about RA.

Create a strong support network. Avoid isolation. Accept your limitations, and focus on what you can still do. Try to maintain a positive attitude. And keep the lines of communication open with doctors, family, and employers.

Check out Carol's Web site at www.arthritis.about.com.

CHAPTER FOURTEEN ❧

The Future of RA

These are exciting times for researchers investigating rheumatoid arthritis. Over the last few decades, our understanding of the disease has exploded, so that many people now are able to escape the debilitating results of the disease that plagued patients of the past. Thanks to new medications, better diagnostic tools, and a more aggressive course of treatment, our grasp of RA has improved immensely, which has meant improved prognosis for patients.

Scientists have no plans for slowing down. Intensive research into RA is continuing in labs around the globe, lending hope to the millions of people around the world who suffer from this chronic disease.

NEW DRUG THERAPIES

In recent years, with the arrival of the biologic response modifiers, treatments for RA have exploded, bringing much sought-after relief to many patients. But even with the improvements, many patients are still not able to effectively halt the disease or to prevent the joint destruction. Many also suffer from severe side effects that can be as potentially destructive as the disease itself.

As a result, scientists continue to work hard in the quest for new and improved treatments of the disease. Following are some of those that are of interest.

Rituximab

This medication is currently used to treat people who have non-Hodgkin's lymphoma. Rituximab works by binding to an antigen on the surface of B cell lymphocytes, specialized white blood cells, and then recruiting the body's natural defenses to attack and kill the marked B cells.

In patients with RA, the destruction of these B cells could play a major role in alleviating the inflammation, swelling, and pain associated with the disease. As you may recall, B cell lymphocytes produce inflammatory cytokines that cause the symptoms of RA. B cells also churn out antibodies, proteins that neutralize and destroy foreign invaders. In people who have RA, these B lymphocytes may produce an abundance of one particular auto-antibody called rheumatoid factor. By destroying these B cells, then, rituximab would interfere with the inflammatory process and block the production of rheumatoid factor.

Research into rituximab and its potential as a drug for RA received a boost in 2004, with the publication of a study in the *New England Journal of Medicine*. In a randomized, double-blind, controlled study of rituximab, researchers found that patients with moderate to severe RA experienced improvements in their symptoms when they took rituximab. The 161 patients involved in the study had tried as many as five other disease-modifying anti-rheumatic drugs (DMARDs) and experienced little improvement in their symptoms.

More specifically, 161 patients were randomly assigned to receive one of four treatments: oral methotrexate alone; rituximab; rituximab plus cyclophosphamide, or rituximab with methotrexate.

After twenty-four weeks, all the patients who received rituximab had more improvements in their symptoms than those who took methotrexate alone. The same benefits were seen again twenty-four weeks later.

Equally exciting, rituximab may be able to help patients with other autoimmune conditions, including multiple sclerosis, vasculitis, and systemic lupus erythematosus.

Costimulation Blockers

Scientists are also investigating a new class of drugs called costimulation blockers. When B cells spot foreign invaders, or antigens, they digest them and present them to specialized white cells known as T cells. But when the B cells present antigens that come from the host body, or self, it is known as an autoimmune response, which is what occurs in RA and other autoimmune diseases. In healthy people, the T cell and antigen do not exchange a confirmation signal known as costimulation, so the autoimmune process is blocked. In people with autoimmune diseases like RA, there is a confirmation signal. The signal then turns on the auto-immune response and activates the T cells to confront the body's own healthy cells.

Costimulation blockers interfere with the confirmation message and suppress the autoimmune response. The first drug in this category is a fusion protein called cytotoxic T-lymphocyte-associated antigen 4-IgG1, or CTLA4Ig. The drug works by binding to substances on antigen-presenting cells and preventing the T cell from becoming active. A study published in the *New England Journal of Medicine* in 2003 found that patients with RA who were given CTLA4Ig, along with methotrexate, experienced greater improvements in their symptoms than those given a placebo. The researchers concluded that CTLA4Ig is a promising new therapy for treating RA.

Tacrolimus

When a person receives an organ transplant, the immune system often rejects the new organ. Tacrolimus may be prescribed to prevent the rejection of organ transplants. Recent research suggests that tacrolimus may be able to work as a DMARD in the treatment of RA as well. Studies found that patients who took tacrolimus experienced a decrease in the tenderness and swelling of their joints.

Tacrolimus works by suppressing T cell activity. The drug is comparable to cyclosporine, an immune suppressant used in patients who have received organ transplants that is already approved to treat RA. Like cyclosporine, tacrolimus increases the risk for infection, and may cause hypertension and problems in the kidneys.

GENE THERAPY RESEARCH

All human beings possess a code of instructions on our genes that determine many things about us, including how tall we are, the color of our eyes, and our predisposition toward getting certain diseases. RA is one of the diseases that has a strong genetic component. Not surprisingly then, researchers are looking toward genetics for a treatment that can stop the devastating destruction caused by the immune system in people with RA.

Gene therapy, as the treatment is called, may deliver a more effective and longer-lasting method for treating RA. Of particular interest is the interleukin-1 receptor antagonist gene, or IL-1ra, an anti-arthritic protein that binds to the same receptor molecules that allow interleukin-1 to seep into synovial cells and set off the cytokines that promote inflammation.

Treatment with IL-1ra would involve delivering the gene that encodes IL-1ra directly into the T cells, which would stimulate the body to produce more IL-1ra. The additional IL-1ra proteins would then bind to the same receptor molecules that IL-1 does, thereby blocking IL-1 and disrupting the inflammatory process. So far, studies done on animals have met with success. Scientists are now looking for ways to best deliver the IL-1ra gene and control its production in humans.

A Nasal Spray for RA

Researchers at King's College in London are experimenting with a gene therapy in the form of a nasal spray. The spray would include a compound called interleukin-10, a substance that not only turns off the inflammatory process that causes RA but also turns on cells that can hold back potentially destructive immune system substances.

IL-10 has been used in other experiments, but never as a nasal spray. In trials, the treatment has caused suppression of the immune system. Researchers are hopeful that administering the drug by nasal spray will provide a more targeted delivery of the medication, without the harmful side effects.

OTHER ADVANCES

Scientists are also working to improve their understanding of the disease. Among the questions they're hoping to answer:

Who Will Get RA?

Experts know that early treatment of RA is the best hope patients have for slowing the progress of the disease and stemming the tide of destruction. Better diagnostic tools that can determine whether someone has RA or is on the way to developing the disease could help toward that end. One new tool for diagnosing RA is the measure of antibodies to cyclic citrulline-containing peptides, or anti-CCPs. Not only are anti-CCPs more effective than the rheumatoid factor test in identifying patients with RA, but some experts believe that anti-CCP may even be able to predict the eventual development of RA in healthy people years before the onset of disease.

Scientists are also looking for more genetic markers that can predict RA. In 2004, researchers with the North American Rheumatoid Arthritis Consortium (NARAC) reported the discovery of a genetic variation called single nucleotide polymorphism that is found in more than a quarter of patients with RA. Exactly how this new finding will help detect people who are likely to get RA remains to be seen.

Scientists are also studying rats with a condition that resembles rheumatoid arthritis in humans in order to better understand the genetic basis of RA. Researchers at the National Institute of Arthritis and Musculoskeletal Diseases have identified several genetic regions that affect arthritis susceptibility and severity in these animal models. Understanding these genetic regions is important because they can help predict the symptoms and severity of RA.

In addition, scientists are exploring the possibility of replacing malfunctioning genes with healthy genes in a procedure called gene transfer. The procedure is being tested in mice and may eventually be used in humans to treat RA.

What Are the Environmental Triggers?

Current research shows that RA is triggered by a combination of factors, namely those in the genes and others in the environment. The impact of environmental factors helps to explain why some people who carry the genetic markers for RA escape the disease, while others become ill.

For years, scientists have been looking to pinpoint the triggers. Studies have suggested that smoking and exposure to mineral dust and vibrations may increase the odds that a person with a genetic predisposition to RA will develop the disease. Research also suggests that infectious agents, such as viruses and bacteria, may trigger rheumatoid arthritis in people who are genetically predisposed to the disease. Uncovering the infectious agents that may be responsible and determining how they trigger arthritis is a subject of ongoing research.

What Role Do Hormones Play?

It's a fact that more women than men develop RA. Indeed, about 70 percent of all people with RA are women. It also tends to develop earlier in women and is more likely to be severe. The risk for developing RA may be higher in women who have never been pregnant and in women in the first year after they've given birth. In addition, women who take oral contraceptives may be able to delay the onset of RA.

Given these facts, it's apparent that hormones play a role in the development of RA and its severity. But exactly how hormones influence RA is unclear, so scientists are working to learn more about the connection. One thing does appear to be clear: RA seems to be influenced by pregnancy. In women who become pregnant, RA symptoms tend to subside. Research suggests that in pregnancy, there are special proteins that pass between the mother and her unborn child, and these proteins help the immune system distinguish between the body's own cells and foreign cells. Such differences, the scientists speculate, may change the activity of the mother's immune system during pregnancy.

Is a Cure in Sight?

As of now, there is no cure for RA. The disease remains an intriguing mystery, but one that is inching toward more answers as the disease comes under intense scrutiny by investigators around the world. One avenue of research that intrigues scientists is stem cell therapy. Evidence suggests that stem cell research may hold the promise of a cure for several autoimmune diseases including RA, lupus, and type 1 diabetes.

Stem cells come from two sources: fertilized embryos that are less than a week old and adult stem cells, undifferentiated cells with no assigned task in the body, which are found among differentiated cells in a tissue or organ. Because these stem cells do not yet have an assignment, so to speak, they have the potential to become any other kind of cell in the body, including muscle cells, heart cells, bone cells, and yes, pancreatic beta cells.

In terms of autoimmune disease research, stem cell therapy would involve replacing the faulty immune cells in the patient with ones that function properly and do not attack the body's own cells. The research is challenging because patients must first undergo intense therapies to wipe out their existing immune systems, leaving them vulnerable to infection for a period of time.

Nonetheless, the findings are promising. In one study, lupus patients were given powerful cytotoxic (cell-destroying) and/or radiation therapy to eliminate autoreactive immune cells, then given blood transfusions of undifferentiated stem cells. Once the newly transplanted stem cells became mature immune cells, the patients experienced relief from their symptoms, went into remission, and were freed of taking immunosuppressive medications.

But stem cell research is hindered by several factors. For one thing, scientists say there are not enough stem cells available for research right now. Although present in adult tissue, the stem cells that are best suited for growing into other tissues are those found in embryos. Adult stem cells face the likely risk of transplant rejection. The problem with embryonic stem cells is an ethical one: Some people believe the use of embryonic stem cells—derived from embryos created by in vitro fertilization—for research raises serious moral and ethical questions, which has resulted in the politically charged debates over stem cell research. After all, embryonic stem cells come from controversial sources, namely aborted fetuses, discarded surplus embryos created for in vitro fertilization, and human cloning.

The successful use of stem cells also will require scientists to find ways to coax stem cells into proliferating into sufficient amounts, differentiating into the desired cell types, and surviving in the patient without rejection. They must devise methods to ensure that the newly transplanted stem cells will integrate into the surrounding tissue, continue functioning properly for the long term, and not pose any health risks to the patient.

So while stem cell research holds the promise of a cure, investigators must overcome some significant challenges before declaring it a viable treatment or cure for RA.

CLINICAL TRIALS: SHOULD YOU ASSIST IN RESEARCH?

Advances in the treatment of RA could not be achieved without the help of investigators. But the research wouldn't be possible without the participation of important people: the patients.

Before any medical treatment can be approved by the U.S. Food and Drug Administration, several research studies are required to prove that the treatment is safe and effective. That's where clinical trials come in. Clinical trials, also called clinical studies, are carefully conducted research studies done in human volunteers to answer specific questions about a treatment or therapy. The treatment might be a new vaccine, drug, medical device, or procedure. The trials are done after research in laboratories shows promising results in animals. The goal is then to find out how the new therapy or procedure will work in people, and to determine its risks and its effectiveness. Clinical trials also look at methods of prevention, diagnosis, screening, and ways to improve quality of life.

Several different kinds of organizations are involved in doing clinical trials, including doctors, medical institutions, pharmaceutical companies, foundations, government agencies, and others. The trials are done in various settings, ranging from a small doctor's office to a large university setting or hospital. All clinical trials are governed by an Institutional Review Board made up of an independent committee of physicians, community advocates, and others that oversee the ethics of the research, ensures that the rights of the participants are protected, and reviews the research on a periodic basis.

As a person with RA, you might consider participating in a clinical trial of a treatment or procedure for RA. By doing so, you might gain access to a medication that is not widely available. You may also enjoy medical care at leading health-care facilities. Some people may feel they've exhausted all other options. For others, the altruism of contributing to science and the development of treatments for RA may be enough to convince them to join a clinical trial.

Before you can participate, however, you have to make sure you qualify for the trial. Some people may be excluded because of age, gender, the stage of the disease, and other medical conditions. After meeting with the doctors and nurses involved in the trial, you will need to sign an informed consent document that says you understand the risks and benefits of participating.

Being part of a clinical trial does involve risks. Some participants might be given a placebo, or inactive treatment, which is used to gauge the treatment's effectiveness. If you do receive the treatment, you may experience unpleasant, even life-threatening side effects. You will also have to endure more frequent visits to the testing site, treatments, and hospital stays than normal. And for all the time and energy you invest, you may also find that the treatment has no beneficial effect on your condition.

To Help You Decide

According to www.clinicaltrials.gov, a Web site of the National Institutes of Health, there are several things you should know before you decide to participate in a clinical trial:

- What is the purpose of the study?
- Who is going to be in the study?

- Why do researchers believe the new treatment being tested may be effective? Has it been tested before?
- What kinds of tests and treatments are involved?
- How do the possible risks, side effects, and benefits in the study compare with what I'm currently taking?
- How might this trial affect my life?
- How long will the trial last?
- Will hospitalization be required?
- Who will pay for the treatment?
- Will I be reimbursed for other expenses?
- What type of long-term follow-up care is part of the study?
- How will I know if the treatment is working?
- Will I see the results of the trial?
- Who will be in charge of my care?

Before you make a final decision, talk to your physician, family members, and friends. Balance the positives with the negatives and gather information about specific trials. If you think you'd like to participate, check out www.clinicaltrials.gov, which has information about more than 8,000 clinical trials being done primarily in the United States and Canada, but also in some foreign sites. You might also contact doctors, hospitals, or health-care organizations for information.

THE FUTURE FOR YOU

The cure for RA may not come in our lifetimes, but already the enormous progress made in recent decades has greatly improved the outlook for people diagnosed with RA. New drug treatments, coupled with a greater understanding of RA, have made the prognosis for RA better than it has ever been. As a result, many people are able to continue functioning in their daily lives, hold down jobs, and care for loved ones, despite the presence of this once-debilitating disease.

Of course, not everyone has reaped the benefits of these new developments. For some people, RA remains a daily struggle against pain and swelling in arthritic joints. Maneuvering from task to task may be a struggle for other patients. Finding the right mix of medications may require constant experimentation for still others. Establishing the proper balance of rest and exercise may be difficult for those who are accustomed to busy, productive lives.

The good news is that the options for treating RA have grown considerably in recent years and are expected to increase in coming years. Better treatments mean greater hope for slowing the progression of the disease.

But waiting for these medications to meet the stringent standards of our nation's research process is only part of the equation and potentially a long waiting game. As a person with RA, you need to develop ways for coping with the disease *now*. Research and the experience of people who have RA teach us that an empowered, educated patient who has a good understanding of the disease can influence the course of his or her illness. By working with a good rheumatologist and learning as much as you can about the disease, you will gain the confidence you need to overcome any challenges that RA may present. And that, in itself, can be very empowering.

PROFILE

JOANN

At forty-eight, JoAnn has lived with rheumatoid arthritis for more than two decades. She plays racquetball regularly, takes an occasional kickboxing class, and lifts weights. She also works a full-time job.

JoAnn owes her management of RA to a combination of Enbrel and Celebrex, a loving husband and son, and a positive attitude that refuses to let RA disrupt her life. In addition, she gets regular massages, takes supplements, and has acupuncture on a painful shoulder. Her husband, a chiropractor, helps, too.

But the early years of RA were not so easy. JoAnn was only twenty-five years old and working in accounting for a small construction firm when she was diagnosed with RA in 1983. Her doctor immediately put her on 3,200 milligrams of Motrin a day and sent her to an intensive six-week session of physical therapy, which helped restore some of the mobility she'd lost, especially in her wrists and elbows.

Like any patient with RA, JoAnn was quickly immersed in the world of modern medicine, with frequent doctor visits, blood tests, and attempts to pin down the right mix of medications. All the medical expenses began to add up, and her employer asked her to drop her health insurance coverage in exchange for a pay increase. "Since my husband is self-employed, it wasn't an option," JoAnn says.

As it turns out, the company was planning to switch to a different, less expensive health plan, and the new insurer refused to provide coverage for JoAnn. That year, after she finished the firm's year-end accounting work, JoAnn was fired. "My boss couldn't even tell me to my face," she says. "He called me in, handed me a letter, and asked me to go back to my desk to read it."

JoAnn was crushed. The job loss wreaked financial and emotional havoc on her life. "I guess I felt kind of overwhelmed," she says. "On top of dealing with a new disease, I had to deal with looking for a new job. I was unsure of my future health, and my husband had just started a business a couple years before. We had also just bought a house."

The bad economy made it hard for JoAnn to find work, and it was more than two years before she found stable employment. Around the same time, she started seeing a rheumatologist because her regular doctor no longer felt comfortable prescribing drugs at the strength she required.

Her rheumatologist suggested she attend a support group for people with RA, sponsored by the Arthritis Foundation. Most of the other people there were also newly diagnosed with the disease. "I can still remember the first night, listening to everyone's story and thinking, 'I remember feeling like that,' or 'I remember doing that,'" JoAnn says. "I also heard a lot of fear and uncertainty about the future."

The fear of the future, especially not knowing what course her RA will take, JoAnn says, was difficult to ignore. "You never want to plan anything in advance because you think, 'I don't know how I'll feel,'" she says. "This is very hard on families, who feel bad if they make plans without you. But it's unfair to expect them to put their lives on hold, too."

Through the support group, JoAnn began to realize that these fears, as well as feelings of being alone and misunderstood, were normal and that openly sharing them with loved ones could help make them more tolerable. "The key is to be open to talking, but not whining and complaining, which just tunes people out," she says.

Three years after her diagnosis, JoAnn began teaching the Arthritis Foundation's Self-Help Course. The six-week class strives to educate patients about the disease and deals with topics such as nutrition, exercise, and the all-important doctor-patient relationship. It was an experience that JoAnn would repeat for the next sixteen years. "A big part of my mission was to educate people about RA and the fact that it's definitely not the end of your life," she says. "But I feel like I learned as much as I taught."

The classes were memorable for JoAnn, who can still recall many students. One woman, she says, attended with her three teenage daughters. One daughter spent the entire session complaining and whining that her mother expected so much of her and her sisters in terms of doing dishes, making beds, and performing other household chores. "I felt so sorry for this woman, and so blessed that I had such a caring family and friends," JoAnn says. "It made such a difference on how I looked at my situation."

Most family members, however, spoke of how helpless they felt in the face of the disease, how they sometimes felt as if they'd been pushed aside, ignored, and left out of their loved ones' suffering. Hearing these stories made JoAnn realize that her own husband, who worked in a healing profession, must have felt really helpless in his inability to take away her pain.

But the biggest lesson she learned from teaching the class—and from her own experience—was the importance of a positive attitude. "Those who choose to feel victimized and turn over control to the disease are the ones who have the hardest time handling life with arthritis," she says. "Others who are sometimes much worse in terms of their disease actually deal much better if their attitude is positive and they aren't giving in to the disease."

To assess a patient's attitude, JoAnn typically started each class with the question, "If you had to describe yourself in five words, would the word arthritis come up? Would it come up in ten words? How long would your list have to be for the word arthritis to be included?" "I feel that if you let arthritis define you, you are defeating yourself," she says.

She was delighted to witness amazing changes in many of the patients who attended her course. Some people experienced amazing attitude adjustments during the course; others remained stuck, unchanged.

Despite her extremely upbeat and positive attitude, JoAnn has had her share of challenges with RA. She had to try virtually every drug for RA—Plaquenil, methotrexate, Arava, and gold among them—before stumbling on a good mix. She's had surgery twice—once on a painful elbow and another time on an Achilles tendon weakened and torn by prolonged use of prednisone. But always, she returned to the racquetball court after her recovery.

Living with a chronic disease like RA, she says, has been like coping with a loss, even a death. Most people will endure the stages of grief—denial, anger, sadness, and eventually, acceptance—which is exactly what JoAnn did. "I've learned that how well you work through each stage plays a huge role in how well you deal with your arthritis," she says. "Moving on and not getting stuck in any of the stages will help you lead the most rewarding life possible."

RESOURCES

Getting good information about rheumatoid arthritis isn't hard, if you know where to look. And chances are, if you were recently diagnosed with rheumatoid arthritis or are trying to figure out how to manage some aspect of your care, you'll be looking for information to help you take care of your health and manage your RA. Fortunately, there are several organizations that can provide you with the information you need. Here are some lists of good resources for reliable information.

Below are some primary sources of information that offer general information about RA:

American Autoimmune Related Diseases Association
National Office
22100 Gratiot Avenue
East Detroit, MI 48021
586-776-3900
Online: www.aarda.org

American College of Rheumatology
1800 Century Place, Suite 250
Atlanta, GA 30345-4300
Phone: 404-633-3777
Fax: 404-633-1870
Online: www.rheumatology.org

Arthritis Foundation
P.O. Box 7669
Atlanta, GA 30357-0669
800-283-7800
Online: www.arthritis.org

**National Center for Complementary
and Alternative Medicine**
NCCAM Clearinghouse
P.O. Box 7923
Gaithersburg, MD 20898-7923
Phone: 301-519-3153 or
888-644-6226
Fax: 866-464-3616
TTY: 866-464-3615
Online: www.nccam.nih.gov

National Chronic Pain Outreach Association
7979 Old Georgetown Road, Suite 100
Bethesda, MD 20814-2429
Phone: 301-652-4948
Fax: 301-907-0745
Online: http://neurosurgery.mgh.harvard.edu/ncpainoa.htm

National Institute of Allergy and Infectious Diseases
National Institutes of Health
Building 31, Room 7A25
31 Center Drive, MSC 2520
Bethesda, MD 20892-2520
Phone: 301-496-5717
Fax: 301-402-0120
Online: www.niaid.nih.gov

National Institute of Arthritis and Musculoskeletal and Skin Diseases

National Institute of Health
Building 31, Room 4C02
31 Center Drive, MSC 2350
Bethesda, MD 20892-2350
Phone: 301-496-8190 or
877-22-NIAMS (877-226-4267)
Fax: 301-480-2814
E-mail: niamsinfo@mail.nih.gov
Online: www.niams.nih.gov

If you're concerned about a complication or a more specific aspect of your care, here are some other health organizations:

American Academy of Ophthalmology

P.O. Box 7424
San Francisco, CA 94120-7424
Phone: 415-561-8500
Fax: 415-561-8533
Online: www.aao.org

American Academy of Orthopaedic Surgeons

6300 North River Road
Rosemont, IL 60018-4262
Phone: 847-823-7186 or 800-346-AAOS
Fax: 847-823-8125
Online: www.aaos.org

American Heart Association

National Center
7272 Greenville Avenue
Dallas, TX 75231
800-AHA-USA-1 (800-242-8721)
Online: www.americanheart.org

American Lung Association

61 Broadway, 6th Floor
New York, NY 10006
212-315-8700
For the office nearest you:
800-LUNGUSA (800-586-4872)
Online: www.lungusa.org

American Pain Foundation

201 N. Charles Street, Suite 710
Baltimore, MD 21201-4111
888-615-PAIN (7246)
Online: www.painfoundation.org

National Kidney Foundation

30 East 33rd Street
New York, NY 10016
Phone: 800-622-9010 or
212-889-2210
Fax: (212) 689-9261
Online: www.kidney.org

National Osteoporosis Foundation
1232 22nd Street NW
Washington, D.C. 20037-1292
202-223-2226
www.nof.org

U.S. Food and Drug Administration
5600 Fishers Lane
Rockville, MD 20857-0001
888-INFO-FDA (888-463-6332)
Online: www.fda.gov

OTHER HELPFUL WEB SITES:

CAM on PubMed
Developed by NCCAM and the National Library of Medicine
www.nlm.nih.gov/nccam/camonpubmed.html

Centers for Disease Control and Prevention (CDC)
National Center for Chronic Disease Prevention and
Health Promotion
www.cdc.gov/nccdphp/arthritis/index.htm

ClinicalTrials.gov
Sponsored by the National Institutes of Health and the
U.S. Food and Drug Administration
www.clinicaltrials.gov

FDA's Center for Food Safety and Applied Nutrition
www.cfsan.fda.gov

Hospital for Special Surgery's Division of Rheumatology
http://rheumatology.hss.edu

The International Bibliographic Information on Dietary Supplements Database
http://ods.od.nih.gov/Health_Information/IBIDS.aspx

Johns Hopkins Arthritis Center
www.hopkins-arthritis.som.jhmi.edu/index.html

Mayo Clinic
www.mayoclinic.com

MerckSource
www.mercksource.com

U.S. Federal Trade Commission's Diet, Health, and Fitness Consumer Information
www.ftc.gov/bcp/menu-health.htm

WebMd
www.webmd.com

Several pharmaceutical companies offer online information about their products and the diseases they treat, including medications for rheumatoid arthritis. Some of the online Web sites for these drugs include:

Arava: www.arava.com
Enbrel: http://enbrel.com/index.jsp
Humira: www.humira.com
Remicade: www.remicade.com

GLOSSARY

Acupressure: A practice similar to acupuncture that uses applied finger pressure to stimulate the pathways of energy and promote healing.

Acupuncture: An ancient Chinese medicine in which tiny needles are inserted into the skin in order to open up pathways of energy and promote healing.

Anemia of chronic disease: A complication of RA in which the number of red blood cells is reduced as a result of long-term inflammation.

Ankylosing spondylitis: An arthritic condition that may be confused with RA that typically begins in young adults in their twenties and thirties. It is marked early on by pain and stiffness in the lower back and buttocks.

Anti-CCP antibodies (antibodies to cyclic citrulline-containing peptides): A substance found in the blood that is used as a diagnostic measure to determine the presence of RA.

Antigens: Substances foreign to the body, such as bacteria or viruses, that trigger an immune response.

Antinuclear antibodies (ANA): An antibody commonly produced by people who have connective tissue diseases such as rheumatoid arthritis, lupus, scleroderma, Sjögren's syndrome, and mixed connective tissue disease. ANAs may also be present in healthy people.

Antioxidants: Vitamins that may counter the joint destruction caused by free-oxygen radicals. The antioxidant vitamins are vitamin C, vitamin E, and beta-carotene, which forms vitamin A.

Arthritis: A word that describes conditions involving inflammation of the joints. There are more than one-hundred kinds of arthritis, including rheumatoid arthritis and osteoarthritis.

Arthritis/spondylitis associated with inflammatory bowel disease: A condition in which the arthritis, or inflammation of the joints, is accompanied by Crohn's disease or ulcerative colitis. Crohn's disease involves inflammation of the colon or small intestines, and ulcerative colitis is characterized by ulcers and inflammation of the lining of the colon.

Arthrocentesis: A procedure in which fluid is extracted from the joint using a needle for purposes of examination.

Arthrodesis: A surgery in which the two bones of the joint are joined together, so that they become less flexible. Also known as joint fusion, the surgery may be recommended when joints become painful and unstable.

Arthroplasty: A type of surgery that involves replacing the damaged joint by rebuilding it, or resurfacing or relining the ends of the bones where the cartilage has eroded or bone has been destroyed.

Arthroscopy: A procedure using a very thin tube with a light at the end to see the extent of joint damage.

Assistive aids: Equipment such as shower benches, raised toilet seats, and walking canes that are used by people who need help in daily activities.

Autoimmune: A condition in which the immune system attacks its own body cells.

B cell lymphocytes: Specialized white blood cells that churn out antibodies. In people who have RA, B lymphocytes may produce an abundance of one particular antibody called rheumatoid factor.

Biofeedback: A technique that uses imagery and/or relaxation in order to control autonomic body functions such as breathing, heart rate, blood pressure, skin temperature, and muscle tension.

Biologic response modifiers: Medications created by living cells that interfere with the sequence of events in the immune system that trigger RA.

Boutonniere deformity: A malformation caused by RA that occurs when the joint in the middle of a finger sticks up.

Bridge therapy: In RA, the use of steroids to control inflammation while waiting for slower-acting DMARDs to take effect.

Bursae: Sacs located between or under muscles that allow for smooth muscle movement and shield the joint and muscle from friction as well as external pressure.

Calcium: An essential mineral that, along with phosphorus, makes up the bulk of the deposit in bone and teeth. In the diet, calcium is available in milk, yogurt, cheese, and broccoli, among other foods.

Cardiovascular exercises: Activities that strengthen your endurance, heart, and lungs.

Carpal tunnel syndrome: A nerve entrapment condition that develops when the median nerve that runs through the wrist becomes compressed due to swelling and pressure inside the joint. If it occurs at the elbow, it is called ulnar nerve entrapment.

Cartilage: A covering at the end of each bone that acts as a cushion for the bone. Cartilage is made up of cells called chrondrocytes and surrounded in a framework of connective tissue called collagen.

Chiropractics: An ancient healing practice that involves manipulating the spine as a way to improve your health.

Clinical trials: Carefully conducted research studies done in human volunteers to answer specific questions about a treatment or therapy. The trials, also called clinical studies, are done after studies in animals show promising results.

Cognitive-behavioral therapy: A type of psychotherapy that works by changing the way the patient thinks and behaves.

Complements: Immune complexes in the blood that become clumps of sticky proteins inside the joint and perpetuate further inflammation in the RA joint.

Computerized axial tomography (CAT or CT scans): Advanced X-rays that shoot several X-rays from different vantage points, and which are then viewed on a computer screen.

Corticosteroids: Medications that mimic naturally occurring substances in the body that reduce inflammation. Also called glucocorticoids or steroids.

Costimulation blockers: A new class of medications that interfere with the autoimmune response in RA.

COX-2 inhibitors: A relatively new category of anti-inflammatory medications that are said to cause less distress to the stomach than traditional nonsteroidal anti-inflammatory drugs. The category includes Celebrex and Bextra. In 2004, the drugs came under intense scrutiny after Vioxx, another COX-2, was pulled from the market because of a link to cardiovascular disease. At press time, the drugs were still under scrutiny for the same reason.

C-reactive protein (CRP): A protein produced in the liver that increases in the presence of inflammation, used to help diagnose RA.

Cricoarytenoid joint: A joint near the windpipe that may become affected by RA and cause hoarseness and difficulty breathing.

Cyclooxygenase (COX): Enzymes involved in the production of prostaglandins.

Cytokines: Chemicals that allow components of the immune system to communicate with one another. Two cytokines, tumor necrosis factor (TNF) and interleukin-1, play a major role in promoting inflammation in RA.

Depression: A serious mood disorder that may occur in people with RA that impairs functioning. The condition is characterized by a persistent sad, anxious, or empty mood, feelings of hopelessness and pessimism, and a loss of interest in activities once found pleasurable.

Disease-modifying antirheumatic drugs (DMARDs): Medications that have demonstrated the potential to slow the course of RA, thereby preserving joint function, reducing—or even preventing—joint damage, and possibly inducing a remission.

Docosahexaenoic acid (DHA): A type of omega-3 fatty acid found in fish oils that has been shown to reduce the number of swollen joints and morning stiffness in RA.

Effusion: A buildup of excess fluid in the joints.

Eicosapentaenoic acid (EPA): A type of omega-3 fatty acid found in fish oils that has been linked to a reduction in swollen joints and morning stiffness in RA.

Elimination diet: A technique in which a food suspected of worsening symptoms is removed from the diet, then gradually reintroduced in small quantities.

Episcleritis: A complication of RA that involves inflammation of the connective tissue between the conjunctiva, the transparent tissue that covers the outer surface of the eye, and the sclera, the white of the eye.

Erythrocyte sedimentation rate (ESR): A diagnostic tool, often called the sed rate test, that measures how quickly red blood cells settle in a test tube. Faster settling is usually an indication of inflammation.

Felty's syndrome: A rare complication of RA that causes an enlarged spleen and decrease in white blood cells.

Fibromyalgia: A condition characterized by widespread musculoskeletal pain, fatigue, and tenderness in specific parts of the body, including the neck, spine, shoulders, and hips.

Folate/folic acid: A B vitamin that affects hemoglobin production as well as other bodily functions that may be reduced in people who take methotrexate. Folic acid can be found in leafy vegetables, legumes, certain fruits, and fortified cereals.

Gamma linolenic acid (GLA): A type of fatty acid, also known as omega-6 fatty acid, that appears to reduce inflammation. GLA is found primarily in supplements, such as evening primrose oil, black currant oil, and borage oil.

Gene therapy: A type of treatment that uses genes to deliver new and different ways of encoding information in order to alter substances and processes in the body.

Gout: A painful condition that results from a buildup of needle-shaped crystals of uric acid, a substance produced by the body and by the breakdown of certain foods. The excess uric acid settles in the body's connective tissue, the joint space between bones, or both, causing swelling, redness, heat, pain, and joint stiffness.

HLA-B27: A genetic marker often seen in people who suffer from a form of inflammatory arthritis such as ankylosing spondylitis or reactive arthritis.

HLA-DR4 and DR-1: Genetic markers found on the surface of specific white blood cells that may indicate susceptibility for RA. The presence of these markers, however, does not always indicate RA.

Homeopathy: A healing system developed in the eighteenth century, based on the notion that small amounts of the disease-causing substance can actually trigger a curative response.

Immune complexes: Clumps of sticky proteins that form deposits within the joint and attract more white blood cells, thereby causing even more inflammation.

Interleukin-1 (IL-1): A pro-inflammatory cytokine that occurs in abnormally large amounts in people who have RA that has become a target of therapies.

Iron-deficiency anemia: A complication of RA in which the blood becomes low in iron, often caused by taking nonsteroidal anti-inflammatory drugs, which can irritate the stomach lining and cause bleeding.

Isometrics: Strengthening exercises that involve tightening or contracting a specific muscle without moving your joints. Isometrics are most helpful during early stages of RA and during a painful flare-up.

Isotonics: A form of strength-training exercise that combines joint movements with muscle resistance. Examples of resistance include weights, exercise machines, elastic bands, and your own body weight.

Joint: The point where two bones meet that allows for various movements. The human body has about seventy movable joints, including those in the hips, shoulders, fingers, wrists, elbows, and knees.

Joint capsule: A covering of the entire joint that is lined with a type of tissue called synovium.

Juvenile rheumatoid arthritis (JRA): An arthritic condition that affects children under sixteen and is characterized by joint inflammation as well as pain, swelling, and stiffness. Long-lasting cases of JRA can result in joint damage and altered growth of the bones.

Keratitis: A complication of RA that involves inflammation or irritation of the cornea.

Leukocytosis: An overproduction of white blood cells that may occur in RA.

Leukotrienes: Substances produced by cytokines in the inflammatory process that promote pain and inflammation.

Ligament: The connective tissue between the two bones of a joint.

Lymphoma: A form of cancer that affects the body's lymphatic system, which together with blood forms the body's immune system.

Macrophages: White blood cells that ingest and destroy cell debris, bacterial invaders, and diseased cells.

Magnetic resonance imaging (MRI): An imaging study that uses a magnet to create vibrations in a targeted area in order to produce a detailed image on a computer. MRIs are considerably more sensitive than X-rays, but also more costly.

Massage: The manual manipulation of soft body tissues that typically involves rubbing, kneading, rolling, and pressing.

Metacarpophalangeal (MCP) joints: The first row of knuckles down from the wrist.

Metatarsophalangeal (MTP) joints: The first row of joints on the toes down from the ankle.

Muscles: Supportive tissue in the body that gives the joints the strength to move.

Needle biopsy: A technique in which a small piece of the synovium, or joint lining, is removed by needle, usually to determine the effectiveness of medications or to rule out unusual infections such as tuberculosis.

Neutrophils: White blood cells that promote inflammation and destroy antigens. In people with RA, these white blood cells settle in the synovial fluid, where they cause inflammation. Also called polymorphonuclear leukocytes.

Nonsteroidal anti-inflammatories (NSAIDs): A category of medications that relieve pain by reducing fever and inflammation, but that have been linked to side effects such as gastrointestinal upset and bleeding. Examples include ibuprofen, naproxen, and aspirin.

North American Rheumatoid Arthritis Consortium: A project known as NARAC involving researchers at twelve different research centers. The project recruited families with two or more siblings who have RA to study the genetic implications of the disease.

Occupational therapist: A health-care professional who helps you relearn how to perform activities in your daily routine so that they cause less pain and pose less risk to your joints.

Omega-3 fatty acids: Nutrients found in fish oils that have been linked to a reduction in swollen joints and morning stiffness in RA as well as other health benefits.

Ophthalmologist: A medical doctor who can prescribe medications and perform surgeries in the treatment of eye disorders.

Orthopedic surgeon: A medical doctor who is trained to evaluate and treat disorders and diseases of the bones, joints, tendons, and ligaments.

Osteoarthritis: A condition caused by the destruction of cartilage in bone that typically occurs over time and with age.

Osteoporosis: A disease in which bones become increasingly thin and brittle. People who have had RA for a long time, or who take corticosteroid medications such as prednisone, are at greater risk for osteoporosis.

Osteotomy: A type of surgery, also called a bone resection, that involves cutting and repositioning the bone in order to improve alignment and compensate for deformity.

Pannus: A thick mass caused by the abnormal growth of synovium cells in the synovial membrane as a result of RA.

Parvo B19 virus: A viral disease that can mimic RA.

Pericarditis: A rare complication of RA that involves inflammation of the pericardium, the thin membrane that surrounds the heart and the roots of the great blood vessels.

Phosphorus: An essential mineral that, along with calcium, makes up the bulk of the mineral deposit in bones and teeth. Phosphorus can be found in virtually all foods, but is most prevalent in protein-rich foods such as milk, meat, poultry, fish, eggs, legumes, and nuts.

Physical therapist: A health-care professional who devises individualized physical treatment plans for patients in pain or who need help with physical recovery.

Pleural effusion: A rare complication of RA that occurs when excess fluid accumulates between the layers of the pleura.

Pleurisy: A complication of RA that occurs when the pleura, or membrane that lines the chest cavity and surrounds each lung, becomes inflamed. This condition occurs in 10 to 20 percent of people with RA.

Progressive muscle relaxation: A foot-to-head technique that involves progressively tensing up different body parts and then relaxing them as a way to control pain.

Prosorba column: A treatment option for people with severe RA. The treatment involves cleansing the blood of destructive antibodies that cause the effects of RA.

Prostaglandins: Proteins in the body that promote pain and inflammation, but that also protect the lining of the stomach.

Proximal interphalangeal joints (PIP): The second row of joints in the fingers.

Psoriatic arthritis: A joint condition that can be seen in people with psoriasis, a skin disorder characterized by a scaly rash that occurs on the scalp, elbows, knees, and/or the lower end of the spine. The skin disease may precede the arthritis by a number of years, or the arthritis may come before the skin disease. In some cases, they may occur simultaneously.

Pulmonary fibrosis: A cluster of conditions officially known as diffuse interstitial pulmonary fibrosis, in which inflammation and scarring of the air sacs in the lungs cause a reduction in lung function.

Range-of-motion exercises: Movements that involve moving each joint as far as it can go in each possible direction, and which enhance flexibility, sustain joint mobility, and reduce stiffness.

Raynaud's syndrome: A condition common in people with RA in which blood vessels in the hands and feet or tips of the nose and ears develop vasospasms in response to the cold or stress.

Reactive arthritis: A condition that may be confused with RA that is sometimes called Reiter's syndrome. It usually affects the joints of the knees, ankles, and toes, and occasionally those in the hands and arms.

Registered dietitian: A health-care professional who is trained to understand the chemistry of food and nutrition and can help create a custom eating plan. The R.D. at the end of the person's name means that he or she has met the standards set by the American Dietetic Association and passed a national credentialing exam.

Remission: The absence of active disease. According to the American College of Rheumatology, remission in RA is defined as the absence of six factors: symptoms of active inflammatory joint pain; morning stiffness; fatigue; synovitis upon examination of the joints; evidence of progressive damage as seen on sequential X-rays; and elevated levels of erythrocyte sedimentation rate (ESR) or C-reactive protein (CRP) levels.

Rheumatic disorders: Conditions that affect the connective tissues in the body and are characterized by inflammation and/or pain in the muscles, joints, or fibrous tissue, namely the body's supportive framework and organs. In addition to RA, other rheumatic conditions include lupus, scleroderma, and fibromyalgia.

Rheumatoid arthritis: An autoimmune disease that causes inflammation in the lining of the joints, resulting in a decrease in the range of motion of the affected joints. The condition also causes swelling, pain, and warmth. In extreme cases, the disease can spread elsewhere and affect major organs.

Rheumatoid nodules: Tiny bumps that appear under the skin in approximately 30 percent of people with RA. The nodules are not attached to anything but are free-floating lumps usually found in the back of the elbow.

Rheumatologist: A medical doctor who specializes in the diagnosis and treatment of arthritis, certain autoimmune disorders, conditions involving musculoskeletal pain, and osteoporosis.

Scleritis: A complication of RA caused by inflammation of the whites of the eyes. It may cause vision problems. Also called episcleritis.

Sjögren's syndrome: A complication of RA that occurs when tear glands in the eyes and salivary glands in the mouth become inflamed, causing dryness.

Splint: A device made of plastic and fabric that helps immobilize a joint and ensures it has maximal rest. Splints can improve function and lessen pain and inflammation.

Stem cells: Undifferentiated cells found in embryos and adult tissue that have not been assigned a specific task and that may be used to generate new, healthy cells.

Strength training: A form of exercise that builds muscles, which in turn helps support and protect the joints.

Swan neck deformity: A malformation in the middle joint of the finger in which the middle of the finger bends down and the joint nearest the tip of the finger bends up, creating the appearance of a swan's neck.

Symmetric arthritis: Simultaneous involvement of the same joint areas on both sides of the body.

Synovectomy: A surgical procedure that involves removing the inflamed joint lining.

Synovial fluid: A lubricating substance produced by the synovium that nourishes the cartilage and bones inside the joint capsule and allows the joint to move smoothly.

Synovitis: Inflammation of the joint lining, caused by RA.

Synovium: A thin layer of cells inside the joint capsule that is also called the synovial membrane.

Systemic lupus erythematosus (SLE): An autoimmune condition in which the body's immune system turns on its own healthy tissues and causes symptoms that may include painful or swollen joints, fatigue, unexplained fever, skin rashes, and kidney problems.

Tai chi: A martial art that uses gentle, flowing motions and deep breathing and concentration. It has been found to improve the range of motion in the joints of the legs and ankles in RA patients.

Target heart rate: The heart rate, or the number of times your heart beats in a given time period, that provides maximal cardiovascular benefits. It is calculated by subtracting your age from 220, then multiplying that number by 0.70, or 70 percent of your maximal rate.

T cell lymphocytes: White blood cells that contribute to the release of cytokines and cause the synovial cells to multiply abnormally, significantly increasing the bulk of the synovium. In people with RA, the most common T cells are the Th1 helper cells, which promote inflammation.

Tendon: A type of tissue that attaches muscles to bones.

Tendon sheath: An encasement around the tendon that helps it move smoothly.

Tendon transfer and reconstruction: A surgical procedure in which a tendon is borrowed from one site and used to replace another tendon.

Tenosynovectomy: A type of surgery that involves removing inflamed tendons.

Thrombocytosis: Excessive production of blood platelets, the substance responsible for clotting, that may occur in RA.

Tumor necrosis factor (TNF): A pro-inflammatory cytokine that occurs in abnormally large amounts in people who have RA. It has become a target of therapies.

Ulnar deviation: A deformity in which the fingers bend toward the outer part of the arm, where the ulnar bone is located.

Ultrasound: An imaging technique that uses high-frequency sound waves to produce images on a monitor. In RA, it provides visual images of inflammation and damage in the small joints of the hands and feet.

Undifferentiated spondyloarthropathy: A diagnosis made when the patient has a mix of signs and symptoms of various rheumatic conditions affecting the spine, but they don't seem to fit in one category.

Vasculitis: Inflammation of the blood vessels that may occur as a complication in people with RA.

Vitamin B6: A B vitamin that may be reduced by inflammation in patients with RA. Studies have found that low levels of vitamin B6 have been associated with increased activity, severity, and pain of RA.

Vitamin D: A fat-soluble vitamin essential for the absorption of calcium and phosphorus; it can be found in fortified milk and sunlight. Preliminary research suggests vitamin D may have a protective role in RA, and may alleviate joint and muscle pain in patients who are vitamin D deficient.

Water resistance training: Exercises that use the resistance of water to help build muscle strength, while providing support to the joints.

X-rays: Radiographic exams used to view the damage to joints, bones, and cartilage that occurs in RA.

BIBLIOGRAPHY

BOOKS

The Arthritis Foundation. *The Guide to Good Living with Rheumatoid Arthritis.* Atlanta, GA: Arthritis Foundation, 2000.

"Autoimmune diseases and the promise of stem cell-based therapies," *Stem Cells Book: Scientific Progress and Future Research Direction,* chapter 6, June 2001, p. 59. Online: http://stemcells.nih.gov/info/scireport/ODFs/chapter6.pdf.

Cook, Allan R. (editor). *Arthritis Sourcebook.* Detroit, MI: Omnigraphics, Inc., 1999.

Duyff, Roberta Larson, M.S., R.D. *American Dietetic Association Complete Food and Nutrition Guide,* 2nd ed. Hoboken, NJ: John Wiley and Sons, 2002.

Goldmann, David R., M.D. (editor). *American College of Physicians Complete Home Medical Guide.* New York, NY: DK Publishing, 1999.

Koehn, Cheryl, Taysha Palmer, and John Esdaile, M.D. *Rheumatoid Arthritis: Plan to Win.* New York, NY: Oxford University Press, 2002.

Lahita, Robert, M.D., Ph.D. *Rheumatoid Arthritis: Everything You Need to Know.* New York, NY: Avery Books, 2001.

Lee, Thomas F., Ph.D. *Conquering Rheumatoid Arthritis: The Latest Breakthroughs and Treatments.* Amherst, NY: Prometheus Books, 2001.

Phillips, Robert H., Ph.D. *Coping with Rheumatoid Arthritis.* New York, NY: Avery Publishing Group, 1988.

Shlotzhauer, Tammi L., M.D., and James L. McGuire, M.D. *Living with Rheumatoid Arthritis,* 2nd ed. Baltimore, MD and London: Johns Hopkins University Press, 2003.

ARTICLES

"1987 criteria for the classification of acute arthritis of rheumatoid arthritis." Online at the American College of Rheumatology's Web site: www.rheumatology.org.

Andrews, Linda W. "Beating the Blues." *Arthritis Self-Management,* May/June 2004, vol. 5, no. 3, p. 14–18.

Astin, J. et al. "Psychological interventions for rheumatoid arthritis: A meta-analysis of randomized controlled trials." *Arthritis Care and Research,* June 2002, vol. 47, no. 3, p. 291–302.

Bjerklie, David. "Rheumatoid arthritis: the other crippling joint disease." *Time,* December 9, 2002. Online: www.time.com/time/covers/1101021209/rheumatoid.html.

Boyles, Salynn. "Diabetes, smoking increase risk of rheumatoid arthritis." September 19, 2001, www.webmd.com.

Cerhan, JR et al. "Antioxidant micronutrients and risk of rheumatoid arthritis in a cohort of older women." *American Journal of Epidemiology,* February 2003, vol. 157, no. 4, p. 345–54.

Chustecka, Zosia. "Genetic marker doubles the risk of RA." July 7, 2004. Online: info@jointandbone.org.

David, J. et al. "The effect of acupuncture on patients with rheumatoid arthritis: a randomized placebo-controlled crossover study." *Rheumatology* (Oxford), September 1999, vol. 38, no. 9, p. 864–69.

De Jong, Z. et al. "Is a long-term high-intensity exercise program effective and safe in patients with rheumatoid arthritis? Results of a randomized controlled trial." *Arthritis and Rheumatism,* vol. 48, no. 9, p. 2415–24.

De Jong, Z. et al. "Slowing of bone loss in patients with rheumatoid arthritis by long-term high-intensity exercise: results of a randomized, controlled trial." *Arthritis and Rheumatism,* vol. 50, no. 4, p. 1066–76.

"Development of a new rheumatoid arthritis 'nasal spray' therapy." Arthritis Research Campaign, July 2004, www.arc.org/uk/newsviews/press/K0588.htm.

Dickens, C. et al. "Depression in rheumatoid arthritis: a systematic review of the literature with meta-analysis." *Psychomatic Medicine,* 2002, no. 64, p. 52–60.

Emery, P. "The therapeutic potential of costimulatory blockade with CTLA4Ig in rheumatoid arthritis." *Expert Opinion on Investigational Drugs,* April 1, 2003, vol. 12, no. 4, p. 673–81. Abstract.

"Exploring the immune system." *The New York Arthritis Reporter,* Fall 2004.

Freedman, E. "Chinese thunder god vine gives relief from rheumatoid arthritis symptoms." National Institute of Arthritis and Musculoskeletal and Skin Diseases, October 2002, www.niams.nih.gov.

"Gene therapy may help rheumatoid arthritis." UPI, May 20, 2004, www.nlm.nih.gov/medlineplus/news/fullstory_17864.html.

Ghivizzani, SC et al. "Gene therapy approaches for treating rheumatoid arthritis." *Clinical Orthopedics,* October 2000 (379 Suppl.), p. S288–99.

Gridley, G. et al. "Incidence of cancer among patients with rheumatoid arthritis." *Journal of the National Cancer Institute,* February 17, 1993, vol. 85, no. 4, p. 307–11.

"Guidelines for the management of rheumatoid arthritis, 2002 update." *Arthritis and Rheumatism,* February 2002, vol. 46, no. 2, p. 328–46.

Hakkinen, A. et al. "Sustained maintenance of exercise-induced muscle strength gains and normal bone mineral density in patients with early rheumatoid arthritis: a 5-year follow-up." *Annals of the Rheumatic Diseases,* 2004, vol. 6, no. 3, p. 910–16.

Jonathan, CW et al. "Efficacy of B-cell-targeted therapy with rituximab in patients with rheumatoid arthritis." *New England Journal of Medicine,* June 17, 2004, vol. 350, no. 25, p. 2572–81.

Klippel, John. "Progress in RA genetics." July/August 2003, www.arthritis.org/resaerch/researchupdate/03july_aug.htm.

Kondo, H. et al. "Efficacy and safety of tacrolimus (FK506) in treatment of rheumatoid arthritis: a randomized, double-blind, placebo-controlled dose-finding study." *Journal of Rheumatology*, February 2004, vol. 31, no. 2, p. 243–51.

Kremer, JM et al. "Treatment of rheumatoid arthritis by selective inhibition of T-cell activation with fusion protein CTLA4Ig." *New England Journal of Medicine*, November 13, 2003, vol. 349, no. 20, p. 1907–15.

Lee, DM and PH Schur. "Clinical utility of the anti-CCP assay in patients with rheumatic diseases." *Annals of Rheumatic Disease*, September 2003, vol. 62, no. 9, p. 870–74.

Levien, TL. "What do you need to know about NSAIDS?" *Arthritis Self-Management*, July/August 2004, vol. 5, no. 4, p. 24–27.

"Lymphoma in rheumatoid arthritis: the effect of methotrexate and anti-TNF therapy in 18,572 patients." http://www.hopkins-arthritis.som.jhmi.edu/edu/acr2003/ra-treatments.html#543.

Mann, Denise. "Occupational exposures increase RA risk." July 5, 2004, info@jointandbone.org.

McCarey, DW et al. "Tacrolimus therapy in rheumatoid arthritis." *Rheumatology*, June 8, 2004, vol. 43, no. 8, p. 946–48.

Mellenkjaer, L. et al. "Rheumatoid arthritis and cancer risk." *European Journal of Cancer*, September 1996, vol. 32A, no. 10, p. 1753–57.

"Nasal spray for arthritis planned." BBC News, Aug. 3, 2004, www.news.bbc.co.uk/go/pr/fr/-/1/hi/health/3528300.stm.

Neuberger, G. et al. "Effects of exercise on fatigue, aerobic fitness, and disease activity measures in persons with rheumatoid arthritis." (Published online Dec. 7, 1998.) *Research in Nursing and Health,* vol. 20, no. 3, p. 195–204.

Ngeow, JYF. "Acupuncture and rheumatoid arthritis." December 14, 2000, Rheumatoid Arthritis Lecture Summaries, www.hss.edu.

Ostergaard, M. and C. Wiell. "Ultrasonography in rheumatoid arthritis: a very promising method still needing more validation." *Current Opinion in Rheumatology,* May 2004, vol. 16, no. 3, p. 223–30.

Ostergaard, M. and M. Szkudlarek. "Imaging in rheumatoid arthritis—why MRI and ultrasonography can no longer be ignored." *Scandinavian Journal of Rheumatology,* 2003, vol. 32, no. 2, p. 63–73. Abstract.

Pedersen, LM et al. "Microalbuminuria in patients with rheumatoid arthritis." *Annals of Rheumatic Diseases,* 1995, vol. 54, p. 189–92.

"Pills, profits and public health." Report on ABC News, May 30, 2004, www.abcnews.com.

Pincus, T. et al. "Prevalence of self-reported depression in patients with rheumatoid arthritis." *The British Journal of Rheumatology,* 1996, vol. 35, p. 879–83.

"Positive data from preliminary phase II study of rituxan in rheumatoid arthritis published in the *New England Journal of Medicine*." June 16, 2004, Genentech press release, www.gene.com/gene/news/press-releases/display.do?method=pr.

Rau, R. "Have traditional DMARDs had their day? Effectiveness of parenteral gold compared to biologic agents." *Clinical Rheumatology*, July 24, 2004, www.springerlink.metapress.com.

Rhee, SH et al. "Stress management in rheumatoid arthritis: what is the underlying mechanism?" *Arthritis Care Research*, December 2000, vol. 13, no. 6, p. 435–42.

Robbins, P.D. et al. "Arthritis gene therapy." *Drugs Today* (Barc), April–May 1999, vol. 35, no. 4–5, p. 353–60. Abstract.

Robinson, HA et al. "Tai chi for treating rheumatoid arthritis." *Cochrane Review*, 2004, issue 3. Abstract.

Smith, Michael. "Genes play a minor role in arthritis." February 4, 2002, www.webmd.com.

Solomon, DH et al. "Cardiovascular morbidity and mortality in women diagnosed with rheumatoid arthritis." *Circulation*, February 17, 2003, online by the American Heart Association, www.circ.ahajournals.org.

Solomon, DH et al. "Management of glucocorticoid-induced osteoporosis in patients with rheumatoid arthritis: rates and predictors of care in an academic rheumatology practice," *Arthritis and Rheumatism*, December 2002, vol. 46, no. 12, p. 3136–42.

Svitil, Kathy A. "Defending the joints—gene therapy for rheumatoid arthritis." *Discovery*, October 1994.

Tengstrand, B. et al. "The influence of sex on rheumatoid arthritis: a prospective study of onset and outcome after 2 years." *Journal of Rheumatology*, 2004, vol. 3, no. 2, p. 214–22.

"The use of anti-cyclic citrullinated peptide (anti-CCP) antibodies in RA." 2003, Hotline article at the American College of Rheumatology Web site: www.rheumatology.org.

Wein, H. "Stress and disease: new perspectives." October 2000, The NIH Word on Health, www.nih.gov/news/WordonHealth/oct2000/story01.htm.

"What lifestyle changes can help manage rheumatoid arthritis? Exercise and joint protection recommendations." University of Maryland Medicine, www.umm.edu/patiented.

Windle, Mary L. "Understanding insomnia medications." 2003, www.emedicinehealth.com/fulltext/44104.htm.

Wolfe, F. et al. "Lymphoma in rheumatoid arthritis: the effect of methotrexate and anti-TNF therapy in 18,572 patients." 2004, abstract of presentation no. 543, American College of Rheumatology, www.rheumatology.org.

"Vioxx linked to heart disease." Press release from Vanderbilt Medical University, Oct. 11, 2002.

WEB SITES

American College of Rheumatology: www.rheumatology.org

American Dietetic Association: www.eatright.org

American Heart Association: www.americanheart.org

Arava: www.arava.com

Arthritis Foundation: www.arthritis.org

Bayer Healthcare: www.aspirin.com

Celebrex: www.celebrex.com

Drug Digest: www.drugdigest.org

Genentech, Inc.: www.gene.com/gene/pipeline/status/
immunology/rituxan

Humira: www.humira.com

Mayo Clinic: www.mayoclinic.com

Medicinenet.com: www.medterms.com

Medline Plus, of the U.S. National Library of Medicine and the
National Institutes of Health: www.nlm.nih.gov/medlineplus

National Center for Complementary and Alternative Medicine:
www.nccam.nih.gov

National Institute of Arthritis and Musculoskeletal and Skin Diseases: www.niams.nih.gov

National Library of Medicine: www.nlm.nih.gov

National Sleep Foundation: www.sleepfoundation.org/features/ insomnia.cfm

Remicade: www.remicade.com

St. Luke's Cataracts and Laser Institute: www.stlukeseye.com

Stem cell basics, National Institutes of Health: http://stemcells.nih.gov/info/basics/basics3.asp

University of Washington Orthopaedics and Sports Medicine: www.orthop.washington.edu

Up-to-Date: www.uptodate.com

U.S. Library of Medicine and the National Institutes of Health: www.nlm.nih.gov/medlineplus/ency/article/000431.htm

Vision Web: www.visionweb.com

INDEX

ABOUT THE AUTHORS

Winnie Yu is a freelance writer who writes frequently about health and is coauthor of *What to Do When the Doctor Says It's Diabetes.* Her work has appeared in numerous national publications, including *Woman's Day, Fitness,* and *Weight Watchers.* She has also written for the Web sites www.drugdigest.org and www.onemedicine.com, and contributed to several health books.

Harry D. Fischer, M.D., is chief of the Division of Rheumatology at Beth Israel Medical Center and St. Luke's-Roosevelt Hospital Center, both in New York. He is also associate professor of clinical medicine at Albert Einstein College of Medicine.

Also Available from Fair Winds

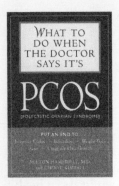

What to Do When The Doctor Says It's PCOS
by Milton Hammerly, M.D.
and Cheryl Kimball
ISBN: 1-59233-004-5
$16.95
Paperback; 288 pages

Do you experience irregular menstrual cycles, unwanted facial hair growth, male-pattern hair loss, acne, unexplained weight gain, and fertility problems?

Polycystic ovarian syndrome (PCOS) is the most common hormonal disorder among women of reproductive age—and the most often misdiagnosed. Often a harbinger of more serious problems, including diabetes, PCOS affects far more than just your ovaries—it affects your body, mind, and spirit. Acknowledging this, *What to Do When the Doctor Says It's PCOS* shows you the diet and lifestyle changes, complementary therapies, and medicines you need to manage this condition today, and prevent the complications of tomorrow.

About the Authors
Milton Hammerly, M.D. is a board-certified family practitioner and Medical Director of Complementary and Alternative Medicine for the Catholic Health Initiatives' Centura Health facilities nationwide. He is author of four books in the Integrative Health Series: Diabetes, Depression, Menopause, and Fibromyalgia. He contributes regularly to professional journals and has taught at the Mind-Body Health Center in Aurora, Colorado.

Cheryl Kimball is a freelance writer and former Director of Chronimed Publishing, a health book publisher with a focus on diet and diabetes.

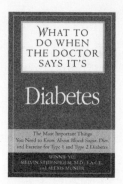

What to Do When The Doctor Says It's Diabetes

by Winnie Yu, Melvin Stjernholm, M.D., F.A.C.E. and Alexis Munier
ISBN: 1-59233-060-6
$16.95
Paperback; 288 pages

The latest research and medical advice for people diagnosed with:
• *Type 1 Diabetes,*
• *Type 2 Diabetes, or*
• *Gestational Diabetes*

In *What To Do When The Doctor Says It's Diabetes*, Dr. Melvin Stjernholm explains how to best care for yourself no matter what type of diabetes you have. Diabetes patients have many questions about medication, exercise, and, especially diet: Is it healthier to eat low-carb? Does everyone have to take insulin? Can exercise be dangerous if your blood-sugar levels are unreliable? How can I take care of myself so that I don't develop Type 2 diabetes? This book answers all of these questions, and explains ways to improve your health based on the latest scientific findings.

About the Author
Winnie Yu is a freelance writer focusing on health and parenting for national publications including *Woman's Day*, *Weight Watchers*, and *Parents*, as well as the Web site drugdigest.org.

Dr. Melvin Stjernholm, M.D., F.A.C.E., is an endocrinologist who has been in private practice in Boulder, Colorado for the past thirty years. He is board certified in endocrinology, diabetes, and metabolism, and holds an appointment as Clinical Professor of Medicine at the University of Colorado.

Alexis Munier is a writer and opera singer who was diagnosed with diabetes at age 13.

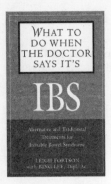

What to Do When The Doctor Says It's IBS

by Leigh Fortson with Bing Lee, Dipl. Ac.
ISBN: 1-59233-074-6
$16.95
Paperback, 176 pages

You are not alone!

Millions of people live with irritable bowel syndrome (IBS). The good news is that there are many treatments, both medical and non-traditional, that can help alleviate your symptoms and get you back in the swing of things.

What to Do When the Doctor Says It's IBS will explain irritable bowel syndrome, explore your treatment choices, and offer solutions that will make you feel better today. Along the way, you'll read about people who have managed their IBS with the unique treatment of Chinese medicine, which has been proven to help IBS. In this book, you'll learn how to find the right practitioner and how to use techniques like acupuncture and herbal medicine to fight IBS and feel like yourself again.

About the Authors
Leigh Fortson has been writing for 15 years. Her interest in health and alternative medicine was sparked when her own experience with IBS was healed by complementary methods.

Bing Lee, L. Ac. has been practicing Chinese medicine since 1986. He was educated at the San Francisco College of Acupuncture and Oriental Medicine, and is a licensed acupuncturist. His knowledge and practice includes ancient techniques that can reveal the source of imbalance, and provide insight into true healing and ongoing health.

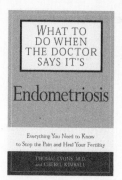

What to Do When The Doctor Says It's Endometriosis
by Thomas Lyons, M.D. and Cheryl Kimball
ISBN: 1-59233-029-0
$16.95
Paperback; 288 pages

Easy-to-understand advice on easing the pain of endometriosis.

Endometriosis affects five and a half million women and girls in North America, as well as millions more worldwide. A painful, chronic disease, endometriosis symptoms respond favorably to a variety of medications and procedures. Knowledge and information will help endometriosis sufferers make wise and informed decisions.

In *What To Do When The Doctor Says It's Endometriosis* you will learn more about:
• Alternative treatments that can alleviate pain and calm symptoms
• How to assemble a health-care team that is on your side and will help you achieve the medical results you want
• The latest research on surgery and infertility treatments in order to make informed, educated decisions about the advice and care you receive
• The truth about endometriosis and its impact on fertility

About the Authors
Thomas Lyons, M.D. is the Medical Director of the Center for Women's Care and Reproductive Surgery in Atlanta.He is dedicated to the development and teaching of minimally-invasive, patient-friendly procedures to physicians worldwide.

Cheryl Kimball is a freelance writer and former Director of Chonimed Publishing, a health book publisher with a focus on diet and diabetes.

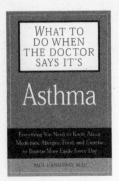

What To Do When The Doctor Says It's Asthma
by Paul Hannaway, M.D.
ISBN: 1-59233-104-1
$16.95
Paperback; 288 pages

A leading expert solves your most common breathing and lifestyle issues.

Asthma affects hundreds of millions of people throughout the world, and every day more and more people are diagnosed with this chronic, potentially debilitating illness. But, with increased knowledge and new medical information, asthma patients can learn to ease their symptoms and enjoy worry-free, active lives. It is important to consider the particular air quality of the towns they live in, what types of medications and inhalers will work best for them, how to exercise to improve their health, and how to react to emergency breathing situations.

In *What To Do When The Doctor Says It's Asthma* you will learn:
• How to assemble a health care team that is on your side and will help you achieve the medical results you want
• The latest research on asthma and new ways to reduce your symptoms
• Alternative treatments that can diminish the occurrence of attacks
• How to help children with asthma

About the Author
Paul Hannaway, M.D. is an asthma suffer and father of two asthmatic children, he has treated thousands of patients with asthma, and has authored numerous publications.